The Osteoporosis Handbook

The Osteoporosis Handbook
Every Woman's Guide to Prevention and Treatment

Sydney Lou Bonnick, M.D., F.A.C.P.

Center for Research on
Women's Health
Texas Woman's University

Taylor Publishing Company
Dallas, Texas

Dedicated to my family

Published by Taylor Publishing Company
              1550 West Mockingbird Lane
              Dallas, Texas 75235

Estraderm™ (estradiol transdermal system), mentioned in chapter 4, The 50 Most Commonly Asked Questions, and the Glossary, is a registered trademark of Ciba-Geigy Corporation.
Illustrations appearing on pages 93, 94, 95, and 96 are reprinted by permission of the Mayo Foundation, from: Exercise and Physical Therapy, M. Sinaki. In *Osteoporosis: Etiology, Diagnosis, and Management*. B. L. Riggs and L. J. Melton III, Jr., eds. Raven Press, New York, 1988.

Designed by Hespenheide Design

Library of Congress Cataloging-in-Publication Data

Bonnick, Sydney Lou.
    The osteoporosis handbook : every woman's guide to prevention and treatment / Sydney Lou Bonnick.
        p. cm.
    Includes index.
    ISBN 0-87833-843-8
    1. Osteoporosis—Popular works.   2. Women—Diseases—Popular works.   I. Title
  RC931.O73B66   1994
  616.7'16—dc20   93-31038
                                                                                            CIP

Printed in the United States of America

10   9   8   7   6   5   4   3

Contents

Foreword

It is a pleasure to write the foreword for a practical handbook that will benefit every woman. Dr. Sydney Bonnick is an authority on osteoporosis, who has spent many years treating and assessing women for bone loss and the predisposition to bone loss. For the last five years she has been the director of osteoporosis services at the Cooper Clinic (a world-renowned preventive medicine center). Recently, she has accepted an appointment as a research professor at the Center for Research on Women's Health at Texas Woman's University. Dr. Bonnick also chairs the American Medical Women's Association's Committee on Osteoporosis, is a frequent lecturer on this condition, and is a good friend.

National interest in osteoporosis has developed on several fronts during the last two decades. In the 1970s it was noted that astronauts lost bone while in space. Weightlessness was recognized as a prime cause of osteoporosis, just as it had been seen in polio victims confined to iron lung respirators two decades earlier. In the effort to protect the astronauts and improve the nation's space program, research was directed at the prevention and alleviation of osteoporosis. Thus the interest in this predominantly elderly woman's disease began as an effort to protect some of our most vigorous people at the time—astronauts, who were predominantly younger men.

In more recent years, we have realized that women in the United States receive health care that is based on less adequate research than the care men receive. Many women physicians, after receiving the good medical education and training that the American system offers, found their training did not sufficiently prepare them to meet the health needs of the women they saw in clinical practice. Many took additional courses, participated in informal preceptorships, and did further reading to fill the void in their knowledge. The public became better acquainted with gender bias in research when a congressional committee investigated the practices of the National Institutes of Health in 1989. As a result of the investigation, the Office for Research in Women's Health was created. A woman, Dr. Bernadine Healy, was appointed as director of the NIH and a massive scientific study, called the Women's Health Initiative, was launched. Osteoporosis is a prime concern of the Women's Health Initiative.

Women's health also became a focus of a new curriculum attempting to teach primary care doctors (internists, gynecologists, and family practitioners) the skills and information needed to meet women's health needs. The American Medical Women's Association's Advanced Curriculum on Women's Health is a continuing medical education course given for physicians of every specialty. Efforts are made to incorporate this curriculum into medical schools, so that all physicians will provide better care to women within their specialities. In addition, the National Council on Women's Health is conducting seminars and courses to increase women's knowledge of their risks for disease and strengths as women.

Women live longer than men, but the disabilities of old age, especially osteoporosis and its attendant fractures, can make the last decades torturous. Women's health and the public's outlay of funds for the care of the elderly would benefit enormously if the prevention of osteoporosis was instituted effectively and universally. Dr. Bonnick's book provides the informa-

tion necessary for women to protect themselves from this disease; it should reach the hands of every woman. While the final assessment of a woman's propensity for osteoporosis rests with her personal physician, Dr. Bonnick's book provides an impetus for women to seek better personal health care. *The Osteoporosis Handbook* will help women become better partners in their care.

Lila A. Wallis, M.D., F.A.C.P.
Founding President of the National
Council on Women's Health

Acknowledgments

I asked a variety of companies to supply photographs that illustrate the medications and equipment used in the prevention and treatment of osteoporosis. All of the companies understood that the use of their photographs was not intended as a specific endorsement of their product, nor do any of the companies specifically endorse this book. Our mutual goal was to provide women with the information and direction they needed to prevent and treat osteoporosis. I would like to thank Ciba-Geigy, Abbot Laboratories, Wyeth-Ayerst, and Mead Johnson for the photographs of their respective forms of estrogen replacement. Sandoz Pharmaceuticals graciously provided photographs of Miacalcin. LUNAR Corp. provided photographs of SPA, DPA, and DEXA bone densitometers. Cybex contributed photographs of their resistance exercise equipment. North Coast Medical sent photographs of several safety devices for the bath designed to reduce the risk of falling. All of the companies provided these photographs at their own expense with no expectation or promise of compensation.

The National Osteoporosis Foundation, Norland Corp., Hologic, and LUNAR Corp. all agreed to the publication of their 800 numbers to allow the public easy access to additional information.

My gratitude and admiration is also extended to the nationwide osteoporosis support groups, which are listed in the appendices. Many of these groups are staffed by volunteers who give their time and energy in the effort to educate and support women in the fight against osteoporosis.

Many professionals assisted me in the research for this book. One is Dr. Robert Heaney at Creighton University. Dr. Heaney's expertise in calcium nutrition and osteoporosis is known throughout the United States and abroad. In spite of the constant demands on his time, he was always a true gentleman and available to discuss issues of calcium and osteoporosis with me. Dr. Barney Sanborn, associate professor at Texas Woman's University and director of the Center for Women's Health Research at TWU patiently explained the nuances of strength training and its terminology and has on many occasions shared with me her valuable insight on exercise programs for women. Phillip Walker, M.S.S., exercise consultant at the Cooper Clinic, designed the basic concepts for the walking programs recommended in this book. His enthusiasm for exercise in the prevention of osteoporosis is always contagious and his concern for the well-being of his patients always admirable. Dr. Everett Smith of the University of Wisconsin shared his expertise in the field of osteoporosis and exercise. Georgia Kostas, M.P.H., R.D., director of nutrition at the Cooper Clinic, repeatedly responded to my requests for additional nutrition information and never complained when I borrowed her books—over and over again. Ruth Carpenter of the

Cooper Institute for Aerobics Research also provided me with nutrition information, as did Lisa Baldwin of the United States Department of Agriculture.

Finally, I can never sufficiently thank Lori Lewis, M.R.T. Ms. Lewis is my assistant and bone densitometry technician. During the many hours required to write this book she kept our office running with little assistance from me. She often took care of my family matters and other personal concerns to allow me the time needed to complete this project; she has patiently and expertly "held the fort." Lori and I have worked together in the prevention and treatment of osteoporosis for ten years. During that time her kindness, compassion, and sense of humor have contributed immeasurably to the well-being of our patients and to my own. Thank you, Lori.

Introduction

When I graduated from medical school in 1973, osteoporosis was considered to be the fate of older women. It was not considered a disease and, as a consequence, there was no emphasis in my medical training on the prevention or treatment of osteoporosis. The only training that focused on problems unique to women was in obstetrics and gynecology, and the emphasis was on childbirth and the surgical treatment of diseases of the female reproductive system. We learned how to deliver babies, remove diseased or injured organs, and treat infections. But no one ever taught us how to keep women healthy. Discussing menopause was almost considered impolite. Nutrition science was in its infancy. Exercise was only considered appropriate for male athletes. Women athletes were forbidden to run marathons in the Olympics because it was thought to be too dangerous. And older women, well . . . older women, like older men, were dismissed to nursing homes and rocking chairs because that was what older people did. The infirmities of old age catch up to all of us sooner or later, don't they?

Only if we let them. In the last twenty years, many of the "infirmities of old age" are now known to be diseases that can be treated and better still, prevented. Heart disease and stroke are excellent examples. Both diseases were once considered unavoidable consequences of aging. Aggressive detection and treatment of high blood pressure and high cholesterol are now accepted as effective preventive measures. Proper nutrition and exercise, along with prescribed medications, are key elements in reducing blood pressure and cholesterol. Individuals are encouraged to have their blood pressure checked and to know their cholesterol level so that they can take the necessary steps to prevent heart disease and stroke.

Osteoporosis, like heart disease and stroke, is no longer considered an unavoidable consequence of aging. Osteoporosis is a disease with well-defined causes. We now have effective treatments for osteoporosis. We also know how to prevent it. Unlike heart disease and stroke, the medical profession has been slow in recommending effective means of preventing osteoporosis to patients. We have been slow to embrace the technology that allows us to test women for osteoporosis and predict their risk of fracture. And, in spite of some very good efforts on the part of the National Osteoporosis Foundation, other organizations, and some individual physicians, we have not yet succeeded in educating the public at large about osteoporosis.

Osteoporosis is a disease of epidemic proportions among women. The National Osteoporosis Foundation in Washington, DC, estimates that 25 million Americans, most of whom are women, have osteoporosis. Every year, in the United States alone, more than 1 million fractures occur because of osteoporosis. As a country, we are spending $10 billion every year to treat the aftermath of this disease. For Caucasian women, who are at greatest risk, as many as 1 out of every 2 women are expected to have an osteoporotic fracture in their lifetime. Hip fractures from osteoporosis may lead to as many as 50,000 deaths annually.

In the face of such overwhelming statistics, how can we continue to fail to emphasize the importance of prevention and early detection? In defense of my profession, I know that I was basically taught to treat disease after it occurred, not to prevent it. But clearly, the prevention of any disease is always preferable to treating it. Effective preventive medicine requires a significant amount of time in teaching individuals what they need to know rather than quickly jotting down a prescription for a drug. Many physicians are already overwhelmed by demands on their time by patients who are acutely ill. The time to teach their patients is just not available. A final reality is that the responsibility for prevention ultimately falls on you, the individual. As a physician I can explain what you need to know and make the appropriate recommendations, but it will be up to you to put the knowledge and recommendations into action. When you are ill, it's easy to remember to take a pill so that you will begin feeling better. When you feel well, it is not always as easy to motivate yourself to follow a doctor's recommendations.

Osteoporosis is also unique because it is a disease that predominantly affects women. Menopause, estrogen, progesterone, breast cancer, and endometrial cancer are all issues that are intimately tied to the cause and prevention of osteoporosis. In recent years, attention has been focused on the lack of research in women's health issues. The social and political biases that have relegated women's health concerns to less important status in medicine have unquestionably slowed our progress.

The Osteoporosis Handbook contains everything you need to know to begin an effective osteoporosis prevention program now. The preventive measures that you can initiate are clearly outlined. The handbook is not intended to substitute for the advice of your physician. It is intended to give you the foundation of knowledge that you need to raise and discuss important issues with your physician regarding osteoporosis prevention. The treatment of osteoporosis is also discussed to provide you with the most up-to-date knowledge of the progress being made in this area, progress that some doctors are unaware of.

In keeping with its objective as a handbook, each chapter can be read independently. I do, however, recommend that you read chapter 6, Exercise and Osteoporosis, at least once before reading chapter 7 or 8, which detail specific exercise programs.

Although we still have much to learn about osteoporosis, we now know enough to successfully prevent the majority of cases. There is no longer any reason for a woman who has not yet become menopausal to silently slip into osteoporosis. For women who are past menopause, any bone loss that may have begun can be detected and halted. Women who have already experienced osteoporotic fractures can be treated successfully, although treatment can be difficult and long.

As a woman and a physician, I have a dream in which a professor asks a group of young medical students what they know about osteoporosis. They think for a moment and then one says, "Osteoporosis. Wasn't that a disease that women in the twentieth century developed, in which the bones of the spine and hip broke more easily? We don't see that much anymore, do we?" *The Osteoporosis Handbook* can help you become part of that future reality. I wish you well.

CHAPTER 1

Osteoporosis: The Women's Epidemic

The little old lady. You've seen this woman before. You saw her in the shopping mall or the grocery store. Perhaps you saw her at the nursing home. She was the stooped, frail woman who walked with a cane. Her back was bowed because her spine was deformed. She walked slowly, as if in pain. If you allowed your glance to linger, you probably thought, "That poor old woman . . ." I suspect you turned your eyes away quickly, too polite to stare and too frightened that, with age, you could become that little old lady.

The woman you saw was not just an old woman. She was a mature woman with a disease—the disease we call osteoporosis. Osteoporosis is so common among women that physicians originally believed it was part of the aging process for women. It is so common among women that as a society, we coined a phrase to describe the woman with osteoporosis that ultimately came to mean any older woman: "The little old lady." Unfortunately, the characterization of older women as little old ladies allowed us to trivialize the effects of a terrible disease. The mindset allowed physicians to lessen their remorse and frustration at the inability to treat osteoporosis because, after all, they could not stop the effects of aging. Physicians had little to offer other than pain medication and sympathy. For women, the phrase

made light of our fear that we might become that stooped old woman.

As a physician, when I see a woman with osteoporosis who is stooped and frail, walking with a cane, I still feel remorse and frustration. My feelings come from the knowledge that osteoporosis is not just part of the aging process. Osteoporosis is a disease, a preventable disease. We know the major causes of osteoporosis in women, we have the technology to find the women who are at greatest risk of developing osteoporosis, and we have medications that can protect a woman from the disease. As a result, my remorse and frustration come from the realization that this woman did not have the opportunity to benefit from current medical knowledge. She didn't have to become that little old lady, and neither do you.

WHAT IS OSTEOPOROSIS?

Osteoporosis is the most common disease that affects the bones. Physicians refer to osteoporosis as a metabolic bone disease, meaning that the metabolism or normal biological function of the bone is affected. The medical definition of osteoporosis is: *A systemic skeletal disease characterized by low bone mass and microarchitectural deterioration of bone tissue with a consequent increase in bone fragility and susceptibility to fracture.* This means that osteoporosis affects the entire skeleton, although we certainly worry most about the spine and the hip. The strength of the bone is decreased because of the lower bone mass or density, which means less mineral per square inch of bone, and because of a loss of the normal internal supporting structure of the bone. The situation is somewhat analogous to not only having rotten beams supporting the foundation of your house but also having a few of those beams fall away because the wood has deteriorated so badly. Fractures or broken bones may occur because the bones are weak and not because of injuries or accidents in which the bones were subjected to a forceful blow. These fractures are called fragility fractures.

This definition is relatively new. In years past, osteoporosis was considered present only after an individual had suffered a fragility fracture. The new definition requires only that a sufficient amount of bone has been lost, putting the individual at risk for a fracture. The definition has changed because of advances in technology. Twenty years ago, a physician generally did not know that his or her patient had osteoporosis until the patient broke a bone. The broken bone or fracture could be seen on a regular X ray. Often the patient could not recall any unusual event that had preceded the sudden pain of the fracture. With a history of a broken bone, which occurred in the absence of any injury or blow, a diagnosis of osteoporosis would be made.

Bone densitometry (also called bone absorptiometry) has changed all this. With bone densitometry we can measure the amount of bone in almost every area of the skeleton. We can detect changes in the amount of bone as small as 1.5%. Our ability to detect all amounts of bone loss has changed the definition of osteoporosis. We now know that a woman is at risk for a fracture when she has lost about 20% of her bone. The more bone she has lost, the greater her risk for a fracture. The new definition also recognizes that osteoporosis does not develop overnight. We always knew that it did not make sense to say that a woman who had a fracture today did not have osteoporosis yesterday. But before we had bone densitometry we just couldn't know that she had osteoporosis yesterday.

You may have heard osteoporosis called the brittle-bone disease. If you could look through a microscope at a bone affected by osteoporosis, you would see why the bone breaks more easily. Under the microscope, normal bone looks like a slice of Swiss cheese. Although there are holes in it, there is more cheese than holes. With osteoporosis, there are huge gaping holes; pieces seem to be missing altogether and others hang by only a thread. In severe osteoporosis, most of the bone is gone. Only a thin shell may remain. It's no surprise that this bone breaks easily, without warning.

OSTEOPOROTIC FRACTURES

The loss of bone that occurs in osteoporosis affects every bone in the body. The fractures that result from this bone loss are more common in the bones that directly support our weight: the spine and the hip. These bones are more likely to break than a bone in the upper arm, even though the upper arm bone (the humerus) has also been weakened by osteoporosis. Wrist fractures are also common in osteoporosis, even though the wrist is not considered a weight-bearing part of the skeleton. If you trip or stumble, the natural response is to put your hand out to break your fall. When a woman with osteoporosis does that, the bones in the wrist must suddenly support the weight of the body. A weakened wrist will break under the strain.

In the United States, more than 1 million fractures occur from osteoporosis every year. Of these 1 million, 500,000 are spinal fractures. Two hundred fifty thousand hip fractures occur annually. Wrist fractures number around 240,000 each year. Fractures of the pelvis, ankle, ribs, and shoulder also result from osteoporosis.

In the United States, more than 1 million fractures occur from osteoporosis every year.

Spinal fractures typically occur without any noticeable blow or other back injury. A bone in the spine, or a vertebra as it is called, that has been weakened by osteoporosis will break during ordinary activities. The break may happen when a woman bends over to pick up the newspaper or put on her hose. She can even awaken from sleep with severe back pain that was not present when she laid down.

Our weight is supported by the part of the vertebra called the body. In osteoporosis, it is the weakened vertebral body that fractures. This part of the vertebra does not break in two like an arm or leg when it fractures—it collapses. This is why doctors often refer to a spinal fracture as a collapsed vertebra. These are also called compression fractures, because the vertebral body compresses. Depending on the appearance of the vertebra when it collapses, it may be called a wedge compression fracture or a crush fracture. The term wedge is used when only the front of the vertebral body collapses. When the spine is

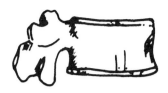

Normal bone in spine (vertebra)

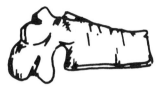

Wedge fracture

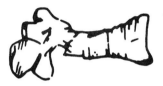

Crush fracture

viewed from the side, the normally rectangular vertebral body takes on a triangular or wedge shape. A crush fracture refers to a vertebral body that is collapsed in all dimensions.

The pain caused by a spinal fracture can be so severe that a woman must stay in bed for 4 to 6 weeks. Even sitting may be impossible because it is too painful for the broken bone to support the body in the sitting position. The pain gradually subsides over a 6-month period. For some women, there is always some lingering discomfort.

With every spinal fracture that a woman suffers, there is a loss of height. Multiple fractures can cause a loss of several inches in height. A woman who was

5'4" before the onset of osteoporosis may be only 5' after several spinal fractures. The curve of the spine also changes as a result of multiple fractures. The spine will begin to curve forward. The medical term for this change in the curvature of the spine is called kyphosis. The slang expression for this curve in the spine due to osteoporosis is "dowager's hump" or "widow's hump." As the spine curves forward and height is lost, the lower ribs move closer to the upper abdomen, causing pain in both the ribs and abdomen. The stomach tends to protrude forward as it is pushed into a smaller space due to the loss of height; the normal waist is lost and clothes no longer fit. Indigestion and a bloating sensation are common. As the curve in the spine worsens, the head and neck must be thrust forward to enable the individual to see ahead. This abnormal posture can cause pain in the head and neck as well.

Unlike spinal fractures, which seem to occur without any provocation, most osteoporotic hip fractures result from falls. Additionally, it seems that the risk of having a hip fracture is greater if an individual falls sideways rather than backwards (useful information if you can plan your falls!).

The term "hip fracture" is actually incorrect. In strict medical terms, there is no hip bone. There are several bones that come together to make up the hip joint. The bone that breaks when a woman suffers a hip fracture is called the femur (the very large bone in the thigh). The uppermost part of the femur makes a sharp turn into the body to fit into a socket in the pelvic bone. This is the hip joint. Osteoporotic hip fractures occur in two areas in this uppermost part of the femur. One type of fracture occurs across the neck of the femur. The second type occurs in the area known as the trochanteric region of the femur. Surgery may be necessary to repair the damage done by these types of fractures.

The tragedy of hip fractures from osteoporosis goes far beyond the broken bone and the pain of the fracture. Half of the individuals who could walk unaided before the hip fracture cannot do so after the fracture. Many women never recover sufficiently to return to their homes; they are forced to enter nursing homes. Every year, 50,000 deaths result from hip fractures. These deaths occur because of pneumonia, blood clots, and other complications from the hip fractures. The complications of hip fractures that result in death are the major reason that falls are the number-one cause of accidental deaths in persons over the age of 75. Falls are also the second leading cause of accidental death in persons between the ages of 45 and 74.

Wrist fractures are certainly less serious than spinal or hip fractures. Nevertheless, they cause significant pain and require a cast or even surgery to heal. Wrist fractures, depending on which region breaks, may be called various names. The most common type of wrist

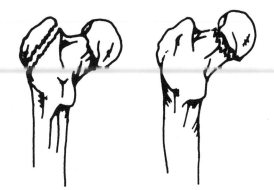

Trochanteric fracture (left) *and femoral neck fracture*

fracture is a Colles' fracture, in which the bone in the forearm (called the radius) is broken near the wrist and the hand is pushed backwards.

WHAT IS YOUR RISK OF SUFFERING A FRACTURE?

The odds are frightening. Medical authorities have been able to calculate the likelihood of a woman having an osteoporotic fracture in her lifetime. The calculations are made in a variety of ways. Scientists consider the number of women of various ages living today and their expected life spans. They also calculate the effects of bone loss on these women, assuming that they experience the kind of bone loss seen in most women today. Because we know how much bone loss must take place before the bones become fragile enough to break, we can actually project the likelihood or risk of a woman suffering an osteoporotic fracture in her lifetime.

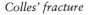

Colles' fracture

A Caucasian woman who is 50 years old today has a lifetime fracture risk of 54%. That means, that 54% of women who are 50 today are expected to have some type of fracture from osteoporosis during their lifetime! The lifetime spinal-fracture risk for 50-year-old Caucasian women is estimated by different scientists to be between 32% and 35%. In other words, 1 out of every 3 Caucasian women is expected to have an osteoporotic spine fracture. The risk of hip fracture is 16% to 18%, or 1 out of every 6 women, and the risk of wrist fractures is 15% to 17%, or 1 out of every 6.

> *Fifty-four percent of women who are fifty today are expected to have some type of fracture due to osteoporosis during their lifetime!*

THE COST TO OUR HEALTH CARE SYSTEM

The costs are staggering. In 1986, it was estimated that America spent $5.2 billion to treat osteoporosis. The money was spent on hospitalizations, doctor bills, pain medications, X rays, blood tests, and nursing-home stays made necessary by osteoporosis. This figure does not include the costs of missed work for the woman with the fracture or a family member who must stay home to care for her. It does not include the costs of hiring individuals to provide care in the home or to assume responsibilities that the individual with the fracture cannot perform.

These costs continue to increase. The National Osteoporosis Foundation currently estimates that the disease costs us between $7 and $10 billion a year. By the year 2020, the costs are expected to reach $30 billion. The costs will increase because the number of older individuals is growing and these individuals are living longer. The actual occurrence of osteoporotic fractures is also increasing, over and above what we would expect based alone on the greater numbers of older individuals. The ever-present factor of inflation is also expected to increase the costs of osteoporosis.

The predictions for future costs and fracture risk are based on the assumption that we will do nothing to change the expected course of events. But, we can prevent these predictions from becoming reality. We know the major causes of osteoporosis and we know how to prevent them. We can find the woman who is losing bone and stop her bone loss. A basic understanding of how the bone grows and functions and what affects it is all that is required for you to begin your own osteoporosis prevention program.

Normal Bone Growth

Most of us think of bone growth as the increase in height or length of the bones that occurs during childhood and adolescence. The ultimate height an individual reaches is the result of his or her genetic makeup and the effect of a variety of different hormones on the bones. In addition to growing in length, the bones also increase in thickness. The thickness of the bone is called its mass or density. The ultimate strength of the bone is determined by this density and not its length or size.

In strict medical terms, mass, as it applies to the bone, is intended to mean the weight of the bone. Density refers to the weight of the bone divided by its size. For example, the mass of one bone in the spine or vertebra, if you could weigh it,

might be 20 grams. The density of that same bone would be 20 g divided by its size. If the size is known to be 16.7 square centimeters, the density is 20 g divided by 16.7 square centimeters or 1.2 g per square centimeter. In discussing osteoporosis and bone development, the terms strength, mass, and density are often used interchangeably.

The maximum bone density that an individual ever has is called the peak bone mass. As part of the normal growth and maturation of the skeleton, the bones continue to increase in density until they have reached their peak bone mass. The length of time that is required to reach peak bone mass is a subject of some debate. Peak bone mass is almost certainly reached by the age of 30. Some bones in the skeleton, like the vertebrae in the spine, may reach their peak bone mass much earlier, even prior to the age of 20. We may have a little more time to increase the density in the bones in the arms and legs.

There are two basic types of bone found in the skeleton. Most of the skeleton, in fact 80% of it, is cortical bone. Cortical bone is also called compact bone. This is the type of bone found in the arms and legs. The other 20% of the skeleton is trabecular bone, which is also called cancellous bone. This is the major kind of bone found in the spine. There are important differences between cortical and trabecular bone. Cortical bone has a much slower metabolism than trabecular bone. That means that the bone cells in cortical bone function, change, and respond in a slower manner than those in trabecular bone. Trabecular bone has a much higher metabolic rate than cortical bone. The faster metabolic rate in trabecular bone may account, in part, for peak bone mass being reached earlier in the spine than in the legs.

There may also be a difference in the response of cortical and trabecular bone due to puberty. The sex hormones—estrogen in women and testosterone in men—may have a more profound effect on trabecular bone than on cortical bone, causing the spine to increase in density during late adolescence.

The function of the bones may also affect the development of density. Both the spine and legs must support our weight but the actual amount of weight that each bears is quite different. How much of a role this might play in the time it takes to reach peak bone mass is unknown.

You may think it is unusual to talk about the bones as though they were alive, but the bone does have a life cycle all its own. It is not just a hard, sturdy framework for the body. The bone remodels itself to provide the maximum amount of strength it needs to support your body. It is continually tearing down old bone and replacing it with new bone. Osteoporosis is the result of disruptions—which cause less new bone to be made, too much old bone to be removed, or both—in this life cycle.

THE NORMAL LIFE CYCLE OF BONE

Within the bone itself, there are living cells whose function is to make or form new bone. These cells are called osteoblasts. There is a different group of cells called osteoclasts that tear down or resorb old bone. This process of bone formation and bone resorption continues throughout our lifetime. In the growing child and adolescent, more bone is made than torn down. As a result, the bone density of the child is continually increasing until peak bone mass is achieved. Once peak bone mass is reached, bone formation and bone resorp-

tion continue at equal rates. In the mature adult, because these functions are balanced, the bone density remains the same. In the mature adult, these processes of bone formation and resorption are said to be coupled. If bone formation increases, bone resorption increases a like amount. If bone resorption increases, there is an equal increase in bone formation. It seems that the goal of these processes is to keep the bone density or bone strength stable.

Replacing old bone with new bone is necessary, regardless of your age. With the passage of time, the bones are affected by wear and tear and must be repaired. This fatigue damage is repaired by an orderly sequence of events that actually begins with the old or damaged bone being removed by the osteoclasts. The osteoclasts actually remove a quantity of bone, creating a depression or cavity in the bone. This cavity is then refilled with new bone by the osteoblasts. The osteoclasts and osteoblasts, which work together in this manner, are called a bone-remodeling unit. The process of removing old bone and replacing it with new bone is called bone turnover.

Osteoporosis is the result of an uncoupling or imbalance in the bone-remodeling process. If bone resorption increases without an equal increase in bone formation, the net result will be an overall loss of bone. Bone mass, or density, will fall. If bone resorption remains constant but the bone formation rate slows, the net result will again be an overall loss of bone. Either or both of these abnormalities can occur, causing osteoporosis.

If the rates of bone formation and bone resorption remained balanced, or coupled, throughout our adult lives, our bone density should remain stable. Unfortunately, this does not happen in the average woman and, to a lesser extent, in the average man.

Bone densitometry, the technology that enables us to measure changes in the bone density, has been used extensively to study bone loss in women and men. Although various research studies have produced slightly different estimates of the total amount and rate of bone loss, they all agree that women lose significant amounts of bone from the spine, hip, and wrist. Men tend to lose less bone from the hip and insignificant amounts of bone from the spine and wrist.

Early studies from the Mayo Clinic, which looked at men and women ranging in age from 20 to 89, found that women lose 47% of their bone density from the spine during their lifetime. The loss of bone from the wrist was 39%. The men in this study lost only 14% of their spinal bone density and an insignificant amount from the wrist. Half of the women by the age of 65, and virtually all of the women by the age of 85, had lost enough bone to be at risk for fractures. Later studies from several universities have confirmed significant differences in the amount of bone men and women lose from the spine, although we may lose relatively similar amounts from the hips. One of the most startling findings from these later studies is that bone loss from the spine and hips may begin much earlier than we originally thought. Several studies suggest that bone loss from the spine may begin in a woman's forties. Bone loss from the hips may begin in a man's or woman's late thirties.

Women lose bone from the spine at a rate of about 1% per year, beginning sometime in their forties. At menopause, when estrogen deficiency becomes severe, the rate of bone loss increases to 3% or more per year. After several years, this increased rate of bone loss does seem to slow back down to about 1% per year, but

6 to 10 years may pass before this occurs. Bone loss from the hip occurs at a rate of about 0.7% per year in women and may actually begin in a woman's thirties. Bone loss in men is slightly slower, occurring at a rate of about 0.5% per year.

THE MAJOR CAUSES OF OSTEOPOROSIS

Keep the definition of osteoporosis in mind: a systemic skeletal disease characterized by low bone mass and microarchitectural deterioration of bone tissue with a consequent increase in skeletal fragility and susceptibility to fracture. What factors by themselves or in combination would cause the bone mass to be so low that the bone becomes fragile?

The amount of bone or bone mass that you have at any point in time is first determined by how much bone you made as a young adult; that is, your peak bone mass. This peak bone mass can then be subjected to a whole host of different things that may cause bone loss during your lifetime. How much bone you lose depends on the number and severity of the different causes of bone loss that may affect you, and how long they last. Your bones today are the sum of all of these different possibilities. In a broad sense, low bone mass can be caused by the failure to develop a healthy peak bone mass as a young individual, by significant bone loss as a mature adult, or by a combination of both. The underlying cause of the failure to develop a healthy peak bone mass as a young adult or of bone loss as a mature adult is an alteration in the normal bone-remodeling cycle. Bone formation may be reduced, bone resorption may be increased, or both may occur.

The amount of bone we have when we reach our peak bone mass is partially determined by our ability to make bone, which we inherit from our parents. As much as 80% of our peak bone mass may be determined in this manner. The other 20% will be determined by nutrition, exercise, illness, estrogen, and lifestyle factors—such as smoking and alcohol use. Although there is no evidence that the ability to maintain the bone mass as a mature adult is genetically determined, many factors can cause bone loss during a lifetime. Poor nutrition, a lack of exercise, estrogen deficiency, illnesses, surgery, medications, and lifestyle factors, such as smoking and alcohol use, may all cause bone loss.

TYPES OF OSTEOPOROSIS

There are different classifications of osteoporosis, which are largely based on the suspected cause of the bone loss. Osteoporosis is divided into two basic categories: primary osteoporosis and secondary osteoporosis. Primary osteoporosis occurs when the bone loss is due to a problem within the bone itself, which causes a disruption of the normal bone-remodeling cycle. Secondary osteoporosis refers to diseases in other parts of the body that also cause bone loss,

making the bone loss "secondary" to some other disease.

An individual can have elements of both primary and secondary osteoporosis at the same time, although one or the other is usually more prevalent. For women, postmenopausal and senile osteoporosis are the most important types.

Postmenopausal osteoporosis is bone loss that is caused by estrogen deficiency. The lack of estrogen has a profound effect on the trabecular bone of the skeleton. Rapid bone loss occurs in the spine and wrist, where a large percentage of the metabolically active trabecular bone is found. As a result, postmenopausal women begin to have osteoporotic spinal and wrist fractures within 5 to 10 years after menopause.

Senile osteoporosis appears to be very different from postmenopausal osteoporosis. In senile osteoporosis, bone loss occurs in the cortical areas of the skeleton as well as the trabecular areas. The rate of bone loss seems to be slower than in postmenopausal osteoporosis. Because there is a loss of bone from both the cortical and trabecular areas, women with this type of osteoporosis suffer fractures of the hip as well as the spine and wrist. The women tend to be about 10 years older before they have a fracture than women

---

TYPES OF PRIMARY OSTEOPOROSIS
Postmenopausal or
Type I
Senile or
Type II
Idiopathic
Adult
Juvenile

MAJOR CAUSES OF SECONDARY OSTEOPOROSIS
Hyperparathyroidism
Cushing's disease
Hyperthyroidism
Paget's disease
Multiple myeloma
Sprue
Corticosteroid medication

with postmenopausal osteoporosis. The bone loss in senile osteoporosis, while almost certainly in part due to estrogen deficiency, is also thought to be due to calcium and vitamin-D deficiency as well as age-related changes in the function of the bone-remodeling unit.

These classifications are rather arbitrary. There are many women with osteoporosis who seem to have some characteristics of postmenopausal osteoporosis and some characteristics of senile osteoporosis. The usefulness of this type classification is somewhat limited. In recent years, even the names have been changed. Postmenopausal osteoporosis is now called Type I osteoporosis. The term senile osteoporosis has now been replaced by Type II. (This was a welcome change if for no other reason than no one likes to have anything that is referred to as "senile.")

Idiopathic osteoporosis is another type of primary osteoporosis. Juvenile idiopathic osteoporosis occurs in youngsters. This rare disease appears around the time of puberty. Fortunately, it seems to resolve on its own after the child goes through puberty. With idiopathic osteoporosis in adults, the bones become fragile and break just as they do in other types of osteoporosis. The difference is that we, as doctors, don't know the cause.

THE PREVENTION AND TREATMENT OF OSTEOPOROSIS

The prevention of osteoporosis should begin with our children. As parents, we need to provide our children with the opportunity to develop as much bone as they have inherited the ability to develop. If we can increase their peak bone mass as young adults, they will have additional protection from osteoporotic fractures in the future.

As mature adults, the prevention of bone loss becomes the most important aspect of preventing osteoporosis. In women who have already developed osteoporosis, the goals of treatment are to prevent additional bone loss and, if possible, increase the bone mass to reduce the risk of fractures.

You can prevent osteoporosis. All that is required is a knowledge of the risk factors and how to eliminate or reduce them. Most of your osteoporosis prevention regimen will not require any assistance from your doctor. At menopause, however, guidance from your doctor regarding bone density testing and estrogen replacement is critical.

Every aspect of an osteoporosis prevention program applies equally well to an osteoporosis treatment program. In treatment programs, doctors prescribe medications that can stop bone loss, relieve pain, and even stimulate the formation of new bone. Research, using new treatments, is progressing. Women who have been bedridden from the pain of multiple fractures can now be successfully treated so that they can return to an active lifestyle, but the treatment can be both long and expensive. The prevention of osteoporosis will always be preferable to the treatment of the disease.

CHAPTER 2

Are You at Risk?

For women, the simple and frightening answer is yes. Every woman should consider herself to be at risk for osteoporosis—it is the reality that we must face. Someone wise once said that the first step in solving a problem is to recognize that there is a problem. You and I must recognize that we are potentially at risk for osteoporosis. A Caucasian woman who is 50 years old today has a 54% chance of having an osteoporotic fracture during her lifetime. That means that 1 out of every 2 Caucasian women who are 50 today can expect to have some type of osteoporotic fracture. One out of every three women is expected to have a vertebral or spinal fracture. One out of every six women is expected to break her hip because of osteoporosis. These fractures cause 7% of women to become unable to care for themselves and 8% to enter nursing homes for an average of 7.6 years. Fifty thousand individuals, most of whom are women, die every year from complications of osteoporosis. This is the problem we must recognize if we are to successfully prevent osteoporosis.

It is ironic that there are those who hesitate to call osteoporosis a disease when it affects so many of us. It has been said that bone loss in women is so common and so many millions of women have lost enough bone to be at risk for a fracture that it can't be a disease. We used to say the same thing about hardening of the arteries. Everybody ultimately develops hardening of the arteries, we said, so it can't be a disease. Now we know that if we treat high blood pressure and reduce cholesterol, we can prevent arteriosclerosis, or hardening of the arteries. An incredible number of new medications to treat heart disease have appeared in the last 10 years. Before this could happen, we had to recognize that arteriosclerosis was a disease that could be prevented and treated. We had to recognize the enormous problem created by arteriosclerosis in this country. Osteoporosis creates a health problem of the same magnitude. It is one that we can solve if we will first recognize osteoporosis for what it is—a devastating disease for which every woman is at risk.

There are women who are at greater risk of osteoporosis than others. The characteristics that increase a woman's risk of developing osteoporosis are called risk factors. When lists of these risk factors are compiled, they are called risk-factor profiles. A risk factor may be a specific characteristic that is known to cause bone loss. It may also be a characteristic that is found more commonly in women with osteoporosis but that does not cause bone loss directly. This type of risk factor is therefore associated with the development of osteoporosis, but is not a direct cause of osteoporosis. There are perhaps 50 items that one could list on a risk-factor profile for osteoporosis. Some are clearly more important than others. It is also important to understand that some risk factors

THE MOST IMPORTANT RISK FACTORS

Female sex
Race
Premature menopause
Lack of exercise
Caffeine
Regular alcohol use
Excess dietary phosphate
Excess dietary sodium
Age
Menopause
Calcium-deficient diet
Excessive exercise
Smoking
Family history of
   osteoporosis
Excess dietary protein

Other diseases such as:
   Hyperthyroidism
   Hyperparathyroidism
   Diabetes
   Cushing's disease
   Anorexia nervosa
   Malabsorption
Medication use such as:
   Thyroid hormone
   Steroids
   Others
Surgery such as:
   Gastrectomy
   Intestinal bypass
   Thyroidectomy

cannot be changed. The practical purpose of discussing the more important risk factors is to identify those that you can change; this will help you reduce but not necessarily eliminate your risk of osteoporosis.

After reviewing the risk factors you can quickly determine what you can and cannot change. There is value in knowing which factors increase your risk for osteoporosis even if you cannot change them; if you know you're at risk, you can protect yourself.

SEX, AGE, AND RACE

Women develop osteoporosis more often than men. By and large, we tend to think of osteoporosis as a woman's disease. Men do develop osteoporosis, but in far fewer numbers than women. Of the 25 million Americans that the National Osteoporosis Foundation estimates have osteoporosis,

more than 80% are women. Being a woman is obviously one of the unchangeable risk factors. What is it about being a woman that makes us more likely to develop osteoporosis? Could we change that? The answer is yes, we can.

Women tend to build less bone then men when they are young for two reasons. Girls become calcium deficient early in their teenage years, depriving their bodies of the most important mineral for building bone. Boys continue to obtain adequate calcium until well into their twenties. As girls, we tend to be less physically active as growing youngsters and adolescents than boys of the same age. Both of these tendencies continue into adult life and create the potential for more bone loss in women than men.

Finally, women are expected to become menopausal around the age of 50. At this time, the ovaries are expected to cease functioning and producing the female sex hormone estrogen. With the loss of estrogen, there can be a rapid acceleration of bone loss, particularly from the spine. Men do not have a similar "male menopause" at which time the male sex organs, the testes, are expected to stop producing testosterone. If men did experience a male menopause they would also experience a loss of bone from the spine, which could lead to osteoporosis.

Calcium deficiency, a lack of exercise, and the effects of menopause are the three most important differences between men and women in the development of osteoporosis, so important that they are considered separate risk factors. Nevertheless, these three risk factors are the primary reason that being female is considered a risk factor for osteoporosis. An individual's weight is also strongly associated with the amount of bone the individual is expected to have. Men tend to be taller and heavier than women, and therefore are expected to have a greater bone mass. This provides some additional protection for men from osteoporosis.

Listing age as a risk factor seems pointless to many people. We all grow older and it would seem there's absolutely nothing we can do about that. Age is considered a risk factor for osteoporosis, based on the observation that osteoporotic spinal fractures tend to occur when women are in their sixties. Hip fractures occur in their seventies. The number of wrist fractures from osteoporosis starts increasing in the mid-fifties and continues to rise as women enter their sixties and seventies. Osteoporotic fractures are not generally seen in younger women in their thirties and forties.

So it seems that growing older increases the risk for osteoporosis. Why? In large part, it is because all the other risk factors have had a long time to work. The longer calcium deficiency persists, the greater the amount of calcium-deficient bone loss. The longer estrogen deficiency persists, the greater the amount of estrogen-deficient bone loss. As we grow older, we tend to become even less physically active than we were when we were younger. The lack of activity increases bone loss. Two other changes occur with age that can affect our ability to absorb calcium. The skin and kidney do not make vitamin D with the same efficiency as when they were younger. This affects your ability to absorb calcium from the diet or supplements. A decline in stomach acid after the age of 60 may also affect your ability to absorb calcium. Both changes tend to magnify the pre-existing calcium deficiency and worsen calcium-deficient bone loss.

These things do not have to occur. All of these issues can be successfully addressed. Age, as a risk factor for osteoporosis, is not as unalterable as it may sound.

Changes that we have not yet learned how to correct occur within the bone as time passes. The function of the osteoblast—the cell that makes bone—appears to decline with age. Under normal circumstances, the bone continually remodels or repairs itself. (Remember, osteoclasts remove old bone and osteoblasts replace it with new bone.) As the function of the osteoblasts decline with age, the bone that is removed by the osteoclasts is not completely replaced. An overall loss of bone is the result.

Other illnesses occur during the course of a lifetime. Some of these illnesses can either cause or accelerate bone loss. Some medications that we may need to take can cause bone loss. The longer we live, the more time we have to acquire these extra risk factors. Again, hidden behind the age risk factor are other risk factors.

Certain races have a much greater preponderance of osteoporosis than other races. Caucasians, Asians, and Hispanics seem to be at greatest risk. In contrast, African-Americans seem to have a low risk of osteoporosis. The reasons for this are not clear.

MENOPAUSE AND PREMATURE MENOPAUSE

Every woman, if she lives long enough, will ultimately experience menopause. Menopause means that the last menstrual period has occurred. Obviously, this is something that is recognized in retrospect. It is not the absence of the menstrual periods itself that increases the risk of osteoporosis. The menstrual periods stop because the ovaries cease functioning. The lack of ovarian function means that the ovaries no longer produce estrogen. Estrogen deficiency causes bone loss to accelerate. The rate of bone loss that is attributed to the effects of "age" is only about 0.5% to 1% per year. Bone loss from estrogen deficiency can increase to as much as 7% per year. A premature menopause is considered an even greater risk factor for osteoporosis than the average menopause, which occurs around the age of 50. This is not because the rate of bone loss is greater with a premature menopause. It is because of the greater number of years that the younger woman is expected to live after menopause. The longer we must live with a skeleton that has been depleted of its strength, the more opportunities there are to have a fracture.

Estrogen replacement at menopause is the most direct and effective means of eliminating this risk for osteoporosis. This issue is one of critical importance to all women. Chapter 4 discusses estrogen and osteoporosis in much greater detail.

CALCIUM DEFICIENCY

Calcium is the most important mineral found in bone. The human body cannot manufacture calcium. We must consume the calcium we need for normal growth and maintenance of the skeleton. Unfortunately, most Americans have calcium-deficient diets, regardless of their socioeconomic status. Calcium deficiency, which is particularly common in young girls and women, contributes to the failure to develop a maximally strong skeleton or peak bone mass. Calcium deficiency in the mature adult contributes to bone loss. These undesirable effects are thought to be a major cause of hip fracture in later life.

In recent years, there has been some controversy surrounding the potential benefits of calcium supplementation in the prevention of osteoporosis. The controversies received a great deal of coverage in the media. The resolution of these controversies did not receive as much publicity. It is clear now that consuming adequate dietary calcium is one of the simplest ways to prevent osteoporosis, regardless of your age. (The effects of calcium deficiency and the benefits of calcium supplementation are discussed in detail in chapter 3.)

. . . one of the simplest ways to prevent osteoporosis is to consume adequate dietary calcium, regardless of your age.

LACK OF EXERCISE AND EXCESSIVE EXERCISE

The skeleton's major function is to provide the framework that carries the body. The skeleton will attempt to become as strong as it needs to be to perform this function. Physically active youngsters develop stronger bones than inactive youngsters because of the greater demands on the skeleton. Active adults maintain or even continue to strengthen their bones with continued physical activity while inactive adults actually lose bone. A lack of exercise increases the risk for osteoporosis by again preventing the development of a maximally strong peak bone mass in the young adult and by increasing bone loss in the mature adult. Regular exercise that requires the skeleton to support the body or resist a force can help prevent osteoporosis. Excessive exercise that leads to menstrual irregularities or the absence of menstrual periods can actually have a harmful effect on the skeleton. Chapter 6 looks at the harmful effects of both extremes in detail as well as the benefits of regular exercise. Various types of exercise are also discussed. Chapters 7 and 8 contain the principles of designing an exercise program that meets your needs.

SMOKING AND CAFFEINE

There are many reasons not to smoke—such as bronchitis, emphysema, lung cancer, and heart disease to name just a few. Osteoporosis is another. Smoking increases your risk of osteoporosis by robbing you of your estrogen as a premenopausal woman. Smoking is also associated with an earlier onset of menopause, and after menopause it can actually limit the effectiveness of estrogen replacement. In all three cases, bone loss can result from the estrogen deficiency created by cigarette smoking. A more complete explanation of the harmful effects of smoking on estrogen and the bones is found in chapter 5.

Smoking increases your risk of osteoporosis by robbing you of your estrogen as a premenopausal woman.

Excessive caffeine from any source can increase the loss of calcium in the urine. Early medical research suggested that amounts of caffeine that are commonly consumed in American diets could dramatically increase the amount of calcium lost in the urine. This would be expected to increase bone loss. For that reason, caffeine consumption has often been said to be a risk factor for osteoporosis. More recent research, however, has somewhat tempered this view. Chapter 5 explains our current understanding of caffeine's potential effects on our bones and the current recommendations for safe caffeine consumption.

Early medical research suggested that amounts of caffeine that are commonly consumed in American diets could dramatically increase the amount of calcium lost in the urine.

EXCESS DIETARY PHOSPHATE, PROTEIN, AND SODIUM

Excess dietary phosphate, protein, and sodium are often listed as risk factors for osteoporosis. All have the potential to increase an individual's calcium deficiency, although they do so in different ways.

Phosphate is the term that describes phosphorus as phosphoric acid combined with another element. Calcium, for example, can be combined with phosphate to form calcium phosphate. In fact, the calcium in bone is attached to phosphate. Phosphate is a necessary and important component of the bone. Why should any amount of dietary phosphate be bad for the bones?

Theoretically, excessive phosphate in the diet or an incorrect ratio of phosphorus to calcium can decrease the absorption of calcium from the diet. Most authorities believe that the ideal ratio of calcium to phosphorus should be 1:1 or even 2:1. In other words, the amount of calcium in the diet should be equal to or double the amount of phosphorus. Finding that ratio in an American diet is almost impossible. The American diet for girls over the age of 15 and women is almost always calcium deficient. At the same time there is an abundance of phosphate in the diet. Most Americans consume greater amounts of phosphorus than are recommended. Instead of consuming twice as much calcium as phosphorus, we tend to consume twice as much phosphorus as calcium. However, most of the research that has shown excessive dietary phosphate to be harmful has not been done with human beings. Two excellent research studies, which evaluated the effect of phosphate on bone health in people, failed to show any harmful effect of phosphate. The concerns would seem to be more theoretical than practical at this point, with one possible exception.

The exception is the growing child and teenager. During the critical period of rapid bone growth, which occurs between the ages of 10 and 20, we would like to provide the best possible nutrition to enhance the child's ability to make bone. Unfortunately, girls around the age of 15 tend to stop drinking milk. When they eliminate milk from their diets, they become calcium deficient. Milk is often replaced with soft drinks. Not only are soft drinks calcium free, they are high in phosphorus. They may also contain caffeine. This is the worst possible combination of events during a critical bone-building period. This younger age group may be the one in which a reduction in dietary phosphate would be most beneficial.

Excessive protein in the diet can increase the loss of calcium in the urine. Unless an individual increases the amount of calcium she consumes, this will make the calcium deficiency worse. Every time you double the amount of protein you eat, the amount of calcium you lose in your urine increases by 50%. Nutritionists and dieticians tell us that Americans consume far more protein than they really need. The recommendation for protein intake for a woman is 44 to 50 g per day. The most concentrated sources of protein in the diet are meats. A lean hamburger patty, for example, contains about 26 g of protein. One-half of a roasted chicken breast without the skin contains about 27 g of protein. With the addition of smaller amounts of protein found in vegetables, breads, and other foodstuffs, an American diet with more than one serving of meat easily exceeds the recommended amounts of protein. Studies performed by the United States Public Health Service suggest that American women consume an average of 63 g of protein per day. A recent survey of women seen at the Cooper Clinic showed an average intake of 70 g per day.

When one considers all the possible risk factors for osteoporosis, it is reasonable to ask how important the role of excessive dietary protein might be in ultimately causing bone loss and fractures. Ranking the significance of excessive dietary protein is difficult, but it should be considered important. Studies have clearly linked dietary protein consumption to the risk of hip fractures.

Studies have linked excessive dietary protein to the risk of hip fracture.

Excess sodium has already been linked with high blood pressure. Table salt, or sodium chloride, is the dietary culprit here. Excess salt in the diet can also increase the amount of calcium lost in the urine.

ALCOHOL USE

Alcoholism is definitely associated with osteoporosis. In an individual who regularly abuses alcohol, multiple problems can occur and combine to increase bone loss and the risk of fractures.

Alcoholic beverages contain empty calories. They have no nutritional value. In particular, alcohol contains no calcium. Many alcoholics consume a large number of nutritionally empty calories from alcohol at the expense of other foods that could provide calcium, and are often deficient in a variety of other minerals and vitamins that may contribute to bone loss. Alcohol may directly decrease the absorption of dietary calcium by damaging the intestinal tract. In severe alcoholism, there may be damage to the liver. In this circumstance, the liver may not be able to make a form of vitamin D, which is necessary for calcium absorption. Damage to the pancreas, the organ responsible for a variety of enzymes required to digest food, may also contribute to the inability to absorb calcium, vitamin D, and other nutrients in food.

Alcohol is also thought to have a direct effect on the bone itself. Evidence suggests that alcohol poisons the osteoblasts, the cells responsible for making new bone. With poor nutrition, possible vitamin-D deficiency from liver disease, and poor absorption of nutrients from pancreatic disease, the alcoholic is at a very high risk for osteoporosis. In the past, alcoholics who suffered broken bones were generally assumed to have fallen because they were intoxicated. While alcoholics do fall more often, the fractures that occur are often the result of underlying osteoporosis and not the force of the fall.

Evidence suggests that alcohol poisons the osteoblasts, the cells responsible for making new bone.

If alcohol can directly affect the bone by poisoning the bone-forming cells, is any amount of alcohol safe? We do not have a definitive answer right now. A reasonable recommendation, based on what we do know is, if you drink, drink in moderation and avoid the daily consumption of alcohol.

FAMILY HISTORY OF OSTEOPOROSIS

The observation that osteoporosis tends to run in families suggests that there might be an inherited tendency to develop osteoporosis. There are two possible explanations for this inherited tendency. You could inherit less of an ability to make bone than another individual or you could conceivably inherit a tendency to lose bone. We think that the ability to make bone, and not the tendency to lose bone, is the trait that is passed from generation to generation.

Medical studies, in which the bone density has been measured in the daughters of women with osteoporosis, have found that the otherwise healthy daughters had lower bone densities than predicted for their age. Studies in identical twins have also revealed extremely similar development of bone density in both twins. These findings suggest that the amount of bone that we are capable of making, all other things being equal, is largely determined by an inherited ability to make bone. Because of their inheritance, members of some families may develop a lower peak bone mass than average. A woman who develops less bone when she is young will be at greater risk for osteoporosis in later life. Because her peak bone density is lower than average, only a small amount of bone loss may cause the bones to become dangerously weak. A family history of osteoporosis is a significant risk factor for the disease.

A family history of osteoporosis should be considered a significant risk factor for the disease.

MEDICATION USE

Many of us must take medications that can have an undesirable effect on our bones' health. Thyroid hormone and corticosteroids (like prednisone) are the most common medications implicated in osteoporosis. Other medications have been associated with the development of osteoporosis as well. These medications can be lifesaving. If you are using any of these medications, do not stop taking them without contacting your doctor first. Because you need these medications, you must be even more concerned about taking the necessary steps to prevent osteoporosis.

Thyroid hormone is commonly prescribed to correct a deficiency in thyroid hormone production by the thyroid gland. This condition is called hypothyroidism. When doctors prescribed thyroid hormone in the past, the blood tests used to determine the appropriate dosage could not tell us if we were giving too much thyroid hormone. The test could only tell us if we were giving too little. Individuals could feel well and still be receiving more thyroid hormone than they actually needed. There are also circumstances, such as the treatment of thyroid cancer, in which a doctor must deliberately give a large amount of thyroid hormone.

In the last few years testing that allows doctors to refine the amount of thyroid hormone given to patients with hypothyroidism has been developed. This test is called a Sensitive TSH. We can now tell not only when we have given enough, but when we have given too much thyroid hormone. With the additional development of bone density technology, which allows us to measure the bone density of patients treated with thyroid hormone, we also know that too much thyroid hormone can cause bone loss. Thyroid hormone can directly affect the bone, causing bone loss to increase. Although we do not know how many people have actually developed osteoporotic fractures from taking too much thyroid hormone, excessive thyroid hormone replacement is definitely a risk factor for osteoporosis. Now most physicians routinely use the Sensitive TSH to avoid giving too much thyroid hormone. If you are taking thyroid hormone and are not sure if this test has been done, ask your doctor. **Do not stop taking your medication or alter the dose on your own.**

Cortisone, prednisone, prednisolone, and dexamethasone are all forms of corticosteroids. These medications are used to treat a variety of different diseases and can also cause profound bone loss. The association between the use of these

---

MEDICATIONS ASSOCIATED WITH
BONE LOSS OR OSTEOPOROSIS

Thyroid hormone
Cortisone
Prednisone
Prednisolone
Dexamethasone
Lasix
Heparin
Methotrexate
Anticonvulsants
Lithium
Depo-progesterone
Isoniazid
GnRH agonists
Aluminum antacids

---

medications and the development of osteoporosis was noted over 30 years ago. Corticosteroids (the term is often shortened to just steroids) may work in several different ways to cause bone loss. Steroid therapy causes calcium absorption to decrease. At the same time, it may cause the loss of calcium in the urine to increase dramatically. Steroids may also directly affect the bone-forming osteoblasts; studies indicate that the function of osteoblasts in patients taking steroids is decreased. The combined effect is that less bone is made and more bone is lost.

There are treatments available to help prevent the bone loss that may occur with corticosteroid therapy. In addition, careful attention to the other risk factors for osteoporosis becomes even more important for an individual who must take steroids. Like thyroid hormone, you should not stop or alter your dose of steroids except on the advice of your doctor.

Lasix is a type of diuretic or fluid pill. It is one in a family of diuretics called loop diuretics. Other members of this drug

family are Bumex and Edecrin. These drugs are called loop diuretics because they work in an area of the kidney called Henle's Loop. Loop diuretics cause the kidney to excrete sodium and water. They also cause the kidney to excrete more calcium. Although it is appropriate to include these drugs in the list of medications that are associated with osteoporosis, their importance is much less than that of thyroid hormone or corticosteroids.

Heparin is a medication that prevents the formation of blood clots. It is commonly called a blood thinner. Heparin is given only by injection. A physician may prescribe heparin to treat a condition called phlebitis. In this circumstance, heparin treatment is generally not needed for more than a week or two. When used in this manner, heparin treatment is not considered a risk factor for osteoporosis at all. There are, however, medical conditions in which heparin treatment has been used for months, or even years at a time, in large doses. When heparin has been used in this manner, some patients have developed severe osteoporosis. The exact manner in which heparin might cause osteoporosis is still unknown.

Methotrexate is one of several anti-cancer drugs that is associated with bone loss. It has been used successfully in the treatment of many life-threatening diseases such as childhood leukemia (cancer of the white blood cells), bone cancer, lymphomas (cancer of the lymph nodes), breast cancer, bladder cancer, and others. Methotrexate has also been used in the treatment of a skin condition called psoriasis and in the treatment of rheumatoid arthritis. Osteoporotic fractures have occurred when it was necessary to give methotrexate in high doses for long periods of time to treat life-threatening illnesses. Under those circumstances, the potential benefits of methotrexate treatment far outweighed the risk of osteoporosis. We do not know if low doses of methotrexate for long periods, as may be prescribed for psoriasis or rheumatoid arthritis, may pose a similar risk of osteoporosis. Research has suggested that methotrexate may cause bone loss by either interfering with the function of the bone-forming osteoblasts or by stimulating the bone-removing osteoclasts.

Lithium is a drug used to treat manic depression, a psychiatric illness in which an individual may be profoundly depressed one moment and euphoric the next. Lithium treatment can result in an increased production of parathyroid hormone. This is a hormone produced in the parathyroid glands (very small glands found on the back of the thyroid gland in the neck). Most people have four of these little glands, which are about the size of the tip of your little finger. The hormone that these glands produce, parathyroid hormone, causes the bones to give up calcium into the bloodstream. In essence, parathyroid hormone causes bone loss. An overproduction of parathyroid hormone can alter the normal balance between the tearing down of old bone and the building of new bone in favor of bone loss.

Anticonvulsants are medications used to prevent seizures due to any cause. Some of these medications may interfere with calcium absorption and the production of vitamin D. While this contributes to calcium deficiency it also has the effect of stimulating the parathyroid glands to increase the production of parathyroid hormone. In this situation, the body senses the need to get more calcium into the blood and parathyroid hormone pulls the calcium from the bone to accomplish this. The end result can be bone loss and osteoporosis. The lack of vitamin D may also cause a second type of bone disease called osteomalacia, which will also increase an individual's risk of suffering a fracture.

Depo-progesterone is a long-acting type of progesterone sometimes prescribed by physicians to treat uterine bleeding. (The FDA has also recently approved its use as a contraceptive.) It can be given as an injection or as surgically implanted pellets. Although there is not an overwhelming amount of proof that long term use of depo-progesterone will cause osteoporosis, there is just enough to warrant concern. This concern becomes even stronger when one realizes that the women who are using depo-progesterone for birth control tend to be young and to use birth control for years at a time. In 1991, researchers from New Zealand reported in the *British Medical Journal* that women who had used a form of depo-progesterone for at least 5 years had bone densities that were 7.5% lower in the spine and 6.6% lower in the hip than other women of the same age. More research needs to be done to confirm the dangers this study suggested, but until more information is available, the risk of osteoporosis must remain a concern if long-term use of these types of contraceptives occurs.

GnRH agonists are a group of synthetic hormones that mimic those normally produced in a gland in the brain called the hypothalamus. These hormones, called gonadotropin-releasing hormones, or GnRH, stimulate the pituitary gland, another gland in the brain, to release hormones called gonadotropins. These drugs have been proven to be effective in the treatment of endometriosis and uterine fibroids as well as other diseases. They work because they actually induce a temporary form of ovarian failure. As a consequence, estrogen levels fall. The effect lasts only as long as the medication is used. During this period of estrogen deficiency, however, bone loss can occur. Initial treatment regimens using these drugs called for the drugs to be administered for only 6 months. Research studies that monitored the effects of these drugs on the bones during 6 months of treatment confirmed loss of bone from the spine. When the drug was stopped, the bone density in the spine returned to the original level after an additional 6 months. Other studies have suggested that the recovery of lost bone may be incomplete. Concern has increased regarding the potential of these drugs to cause significant bone loss that might not be completely reversible because many physicians are now using these drugs for longer periods of time or for multiple 6-month courses of therapy.

Isoniazid or INH is one of the drugs commonly used to treat tuberculosis. It is often listed as a drug that may increase the risk of osteoporosis because it can cause an increase in the amount of calcium lost in the urine on a daily basis.

The chronic use of aluminum-containing antacids can also have a detrimental effect on the bone. Aluminum can decrease the absorption of calcium and phosphate from the diet and increase calcium losses in the urine. Occasional use of aluminum-containing antacids is not thought to be a risk factor for osteoporosis.

SURGERY

Certain types of surgery may increase your risk of osteoporosis. Gastrectomy, or the surgical removal of the stomach, has been associated with osteoporosis. In one study, the risk of hip fractures was more than doubled in patients who had undergone a gastrectomy. Bone-mass measurements in patients who have had a gastrectomy have documented bone loss from the spine and hip. The mechanism by which gastrectomy might cause bone loss is not clear. There is speculation that both the absorption of calcium and vitamin D may be impaired.

There may also be an increase in the production of parathyroid hormone that may accelerate bone loss. In the past, intestinal bypass surgery was performed to control severe and life-threatening obesity. Much like gastrectomy, the body's ability to absorb nutrients, like calcium and vitamin D, is altered after this surgery. Unless corrected, osteoporosis and osteomalacia can result.

Thyroidectomy, or the surgical removal of the thyroid gland has also been associated with osteoporosis. The thyroid gland may be surgically removed for the treatment of hyperthyroidism or thyroid cancer. In addition to thyroid hormone, the thyroid gland also makes a hormone called calcitonin. Calcitonin is a bone hormone that stops bone loss. When the thyroid gland is completely removed, the blood levels of calcitonin fall. There is speculation that this lack of calcitonin could lead to increased bone loss and osteoporosis.

OTHER DISEASES

Many diseases can cause bone loss, in addition to the other effects they may have on the body. These diseases are considered to be causes of secondary osteoporosis (remember, the term primary osteoporosis is reserved for osteoporosis caused by estrogen deficiency, calcium deficiency, and age-related causes of bone loss). One could also call these diseases causes of secondary osteoporosis because the osteoporosis is, in a sense, secondary in importance to the other effects of the disease.

Hyperthyroidism, which refers to a condition in which the thyroid gland produces too much thyroid hormone, is associated with osteoporosis. The mechanism is the same as occurs in an individual who takes too much thyroid hormone: too much thyroid hormone, whether it comes from the thyroid gland or a pill, can cause bone loss.

Hyperparathyroidism is a condition in which one or more of the parathyroid glands in the neck becomes overactive. Excessive amounts of parathyroid hormone are produced, causing bone loss. The loss of bone in hyperparathyroidism may be greatest in the hip.

Diabetes is often listed as a risk factor for osteoporosis. This is mildly controversial. Early studies suggested an increase in the number of osteoporotic fractures in patients with diabetes, but more recent studies have been unable to demonstrate bone loss or osteoporotic fractures in patients who have what is called noninsulin-dependent diabetes. In general, physicians no longer consider noninsulin-dependent diabetes to be a risk factor for osteoporosis. Insulin-dependent diabetes may indeed be a risk factor for osteoporosis. Studies have shown that these patients will have some bone loss as compared to individuals of the same age who do not have diabetes.

Cushing's disease, or Cushing's syndrome, is a condition in which cortisone is overproduced by the adrenal glands. (These are small glands, which sit on top of each kidney.) The adrenal glands must produce cortisone to sustain life. Excessive amounts of cortisone can cause severe osteoporosis, particularly in the spine. This is similar to the situation caused by the treatment of other diseases with corticosteroids.

Anorexia nervosa is an eating disorder that is all too common in young women. Women in their twenties can suffer osteoporotic spinal fractures because of the malnutrition and estrogen deficiency that results from this disease.

Malabsorption is a condition in which the intestinal tract is damaged, making the absorption of vitamins, minerals, and other nutrients difficult or impossible. There are a number of different diseases that can cause malabsorption; two of the more common ones are Crohn's disease and sprue.

ARE YOU AT RISK?

I hope, after reviewing the list of risk factors, that you have not found many that apply to you. Undoubtedly, you will have found some. Some of these risk factors cannot be changed. Ultimately, we will all become menopausal and grow older. On the other hand, we do not have to become estrogen-deficient and we do not have to become inactive. We cannot change our inheritance or our family history. We can, however, actively protect ourselves from bone loss.

You can change many risk factors. You can correct calcium deficiency and alter your lifestyle to include more exercise. You can avoid cigarette smoking and excessive use of caffeine and alcohol.

The use of medications and the occurrence of diseases that can contribute to the development of osteoporosis may be unavoidable. If these things occur, there are additional preventive measures you and your doctor can take if only the need for them is recognized. A little knowledge is a lot of power in preventing osteoporosis.

Calcium, estrogen, exercise, and smoking are so important that they deserve more extensive discussion. Caffeine consumption warrants a second look as well, in order to clarify the new information about its link to the risk of osteoporosis.

CHAPTER 3

The Importance of Calcium

Several years ago, the banner headline on an issue of *Newsweek* was "Calcium." In bold letters, the cover asked "Do these miracle minerals work?" The article discussed what was known and what was only speculative regarding the various claims made for calcium in the maintenance of good health and the prevention of disease. You and I know that calcium is not a miracle cure for all that ails us; it is simply a mineral. But it is an extraordinarily important mineral, particularly for the health of the skeleton.

Calcium, by itself, is a soft, silvery white metallic substance. It is found in nature in a variety of forms. In oyster shells, a form of calcium known as calcium carbonate can be found. In limestone rock, calcium is present as calcium carbonate. Calcium carbonate is also found in marble and chalk. The chemical nature of calcium is such that it is always "attached" to something else. In the cases I just mentioned, calcium is attached to carbonate. When calcium is attached to another chemical compound, it is referred to as a calcium salt—not to be confused with table salt, which is sodium chloride. Calcium also occurs naturally in milk and other dairy products. In these substances, calcium is attached to phosphate and is known as calcium phosphate.

There are other forms of calcium as well, although these do not occur in nature and must be manufactured by man.

These are calcium salts, such as calcium citrate, calcium citrate malate, calcium chloride, calcium lactate, and calcium gluconate. The body, and particularly the skeleton, is concerned primarily with the calcium itself, or "elemental" calcium as it is called, and is much less concerned with the type of calcium salt. The type of calcium salt may affect how easily the calcium is absorbed by our bodies and the types of side effects that may occur.

Of all the calcium found in your body, 99% is found in the skeleton. The other 1% is in the bloodstream and cells of other organ systems. Within the bones, calcium and another mineral, called phosphate, form the crystalline latticework structure of the bone called hydroxyapatite. It is this crystalline structure that gives the bone its strength.

So how much calcium do we need and how do we get it? What happens to calcium once it enters the body? And why is calcium so important in the prevention of osteoporosis?

CALCIUM'S ROLE IN THE PREVENTION OF OSTEOPOROSIS

There are two basic approaches to the prevention of osteoporosis. The first is to build as much bone as possible when you are young. The second is to prevent bone loss as a mature adult. Calcium is critical to achieving both goals.

With the advances in bone-density technology, the technology that allows us to measure the bone density or strength, it has finally become possible to safely study the development of children's bones, without exposing them to excessive radiation. While common sense told us that adequate calcium was important for developing a strong bone mass in the growing adolescent, medical research has now proved it.

The term "peak bone mass" does not refer to the maximum height that an individual reaches, but instead to the maximum density of bone that an individual develops. While there is still some argument in medical circles as to the exact age at which peak bone mass is reached, most authorities agree that 90% or more of an individual's peak bone mass is reached by the age of 20. The peak bone mass that a child develops is partially determined by the inherited ability to make bone. It is also determined by the child's calcium intake and exercise level. Exercise will be discussed in chapter 6.

Studies that have examined the relationship between calcium intake and bone density in children have found that there is a strong relationship. The greater the children's calcium intake, the greater bone density or peak bone mass they develop. An important study from the University of Indiana actually looked at the bone mass development of 22 sets of identical twins. In this study, one twin received an average of 908 mg of calcium daily from the diet. The other twin was given a calcium supplement in addition to the dietary calcium, increasing the total amount of calcium to an average of 1,612 mg a day. Even though both twins inherited the same ability to make bone, the twin that received the greater amount of calcium developed a higher bone density. The results of this study suggested that not only was an adequate calcium intake important in developing bone but that perhaps we should be giving children even more calcium than is currently recommended.

The development of a good peak bone mass has been strongly tied to the prevention of hip fracture in later life. In a research study considered to be one of the most important of its kind, Dr. Velimir Matkovic and his colleagues investigated the relationship between calcium intake and the occurrence of hip fracture in two regions of Yugoslavia. In one region, where the dietary calcium intake was high, the individuals had developed a greater peak bone mass. In the other region, the dietary calcium intake was much less and not surprisingly, these people tended to have a lower peak bone mass. The number of hip fractures was much greater in the low-calcium-intake region. One of the conclusions from this study was that the development of a greater peak bone mass offered protection from the future development of hip fracture.

After peak bone mass is reached, bone loss must be avoided to prevent osteoporosis. Calcium's role here has generated more controversy than any other topic associated with osteoporosis prevention. Common sense again told us that if the body's daily calcium needs were not met by the diet, the body would take calcium from the bones to meet its needs, causing bone loss. This was difficult to prove because there are so many things that can and do cause bone loss in adults. It was very difficult to single out the effects of calcium deficiency and separate them from the effects of smoking, drinking, lack of exercise, hormone deficiency, illness, and medications that can cause bone loss. Once research was completed on calcium supplementation's effect on bone loss, it became clear that adequate calcium in adults did slow bone loss.

Calcium's greatest benefit for adults may be its role in slowing bone loss from the hip and preventing hip fractures. In 1973, Drs. Troy Holbrook and Elizabeth Barrett-Connor began a study of almost 1,000 men and women from California. The men and women ranged in age from 50 to 79. At the beginning of the study, the average amount of calcium each individual consumed was recorded by a dietician. The men and women were followed by the researchers for 14 years. At the end of the study, they were divided into three groups, based on the amount of calcium they consumed: a low-calcium group, a midrange-calcium group, and a high-calcium group. The men and women in the high-calcium group had the fewest hip fractures during the 14-year study while those in the low-calcium group had the greatest number of hip fractures. The doctors could find no other explanation for the apparent protection from hip fractures of the members of the high-calcium group other than the amount of calcium they consumed.

> *Calcium's greatest benefit for adults may be its role in slowing bone loss from the hip and preventing hip fractures.*

The ability of calcium supplementation to stop calcium-deficient bone loss appears to be indefinite. That is, there is no upper age limit when calcium would not be expected to have this effect. So even if you have passed the age that calcium supplementation can improve your peak bone mass, it is never too late to stop calcium-deficient bone loss with calcium supplements.

> *. . . it is never too late to stop calcium-deficient bone loss with calcium supplements.*

HOW CAN WE GET THE CALCIUM WE NEED?

Calcium is not made within the human body. Calcium is found in nature in oyster shells and limestone rock. Fruits and vegetables contain small amounts of calcium. Within the animal kingdom, calcium is found in high concentrations in the milk of dairy cows and other milk-producing animals. For the human body to obtain the calcium it needs for growth of the skeleton and proper function of other organs, the calcium must be consumed from one of these sources.

See the appendices for a list of the calcium content of customary servings of foods in American diets. A quick review of this list reveals that the only concentrated sources of calcium that are common in our diet are foods from the dairy-product family. An 8-ounce glass of 2% milk for example, contains 297 mg of calcium. A cup of yogurt contains over 400 mg. Unfortunately, two slices of wheat bread only contain 40 mg. A medium-sized orange supplies about 50 mg. Three ounces of a - T-bone steak contain only 6 mg of calcium.

The Public Health Service and the United States Department of Agriculture (USDA) periodically survey the American public to determine the types of foods we regularly eat and their nutritional content. The surveys that have examined the types of foods we get our calcium from confirm that we rely on dairy products for our calcium. This is not so much a matter of choice as it is a matter of necessity. Even with a balanced diet, other food sources do not supply sufficient calcium to meet our daily needs. When surveys were done to look at the types of dairy products Americans relied on to supply calcium, it became clear that the bulk of dietary calcium came from beverage milk; that is, the glass of milk our mothers always insisted that we drink when we were children.

When you look at the USDA graph it is not too difficult to imagine what happens to the amount of calcium in the diet when the beverage milk is removed—the total amount of calcium consumed falls by almost 40%. In fact, that is exactly what happens to most American men and women. Another graph from the same survey illustrates how the consumption of beverage milk drops dramatically for girls around the age of 15 and for boys between the ages of 20 and 25. We stop drinking milk and start drinking tea, coffee, soft drinks, or even alcoholic beverages in its place. None of these beverages contains any calcium.

The Health and Nutrition Examination Surveys performed by the Public Health Service between 1971 and 1974 (HANES I) and 1976 and 1980 (HANES II) confirmed a virtual epidemic of calcium-deficient diets in the United States. The surveys found that after the age of 15, more than 50% of American women consumed less than half of the recommended daily allowance for calcium. During the critical years of late adolescence and early adulthood, when bone strength grows, more than two-thirds of all American women consumed less than the recommended amount.

Dietary calcium deficiency was not limited to the young. The surveys found

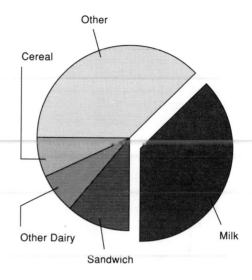

Source: the USDA's Food Consumption Survey, 1977.

Calcium Sources in the American Diet

that 25% of all American women consumed less than 300 mg of calcium per day. Both studies also confirmed that American men maintained a higher calcium intake throughout their lives with 60% to 70% of men consuming an amount of calcium that was actually greater than the recommended amount. Why? Men continued to drink beverage milk longer than most women. They also tended to consume more calories overall, obtaining more calcium from other dietary sources.

This calcium deficiency is not new. As early as 1955, surveys from the USDA listed calcium as one of the critical dietary nutrients commonly found below recommended levels in American women's diets. You might wonder, with all the new information and publicity about calcium and osteoporosis, if this dismal situation has improved by now.

Only a little. In 1985, information from the USDA indicated that women between the ages of 19 and 50 consumed an average of 624 mg of calcium a day. In 1987, women between the ages of 20 and

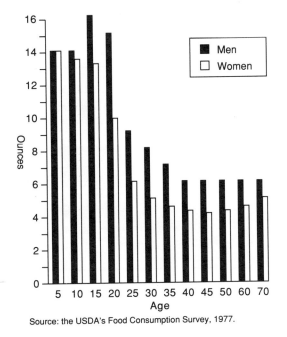

Source: the USDA's Food Consumption Survey, 1977.

Ounces of Beverage Milk Consumed Daily

80 were consuming 602 mg per day but the basic trend in calcium consumption, noted so long ago, has continued. Dietary calcium intake among women falls in the early teenage years and continues to remain low during adult life.

In 1992, the results of a *Prevention* readers' survey emphasized our failure to appreciate the importance of calcium in the diet. *Prevention* asked its readers if the desire to prevent osteoporosis affected their eating habits. In this group of women, who are presumed to be highly motivated to prevent disease, only 65% responded yes to this question. When the women in this survey were asked if they consumed more dairy products and other calcium-rich foods, only 22% said yes! In the 1991 National Osteoporosis Foundation Gallup Survey of 750 women between the ages of 45 and 75 in the United States, 4 out of every 5 women surveyed indicated that they thought a poor diet increased the chances of developing osteoporosis. In fact, 1 out of every 3 women in this survey thought that calcium could cure osteoporosis! That unfortunately isn't true, but if we do understand that calcium is so very important, why do we remain calcium deficient?

Part of the difficulty is that we need so much calcium from the diet to make up for the fact that our bodies absorb calcium inefficiently. The body itself actually needs much less calcium than we recommend that you consume. Let me explain.

Let's assume that you eat a diet that provides you with 1,000 mg of elemental calcium every day. From that 1,000 mg, your body only absorbs 25%, or 250 milligrams. Sometimes it does a little better and sometimes it actually doesn't do as well. But for the moment, let's say that only 250 mg of that 1,000 mg that you ate actually makes it into the bloodstream. In the meantime, your bloodstream is sending back, or secreting into the intestinal tract, about 100 mg of calcium. This is added to the calcium that you did not absorb from the food and is lost from the body as part of the stool. Of the 250 mg you absorbed, about 150 mg is taken from the blood by the kidneys and passed into the urine. These losses of calcium into the stool and urine are called obligatory losses. That means that they will occur regardless of the amount of calcium we actually consume. The body's actual goal in all of this is to keep the level of calcium in the blood constant. So if we don't consume enough calcium to keep up with the losses of calcium into the urine and stool, the blood calcium will fall unless the body replaces the blood calcium from another source. In its infinite wisdom, that is exactly what the body does. We would otherwise die. Unfortunately, the body's reserve source of calcium is the bones.

How Much Calcium Do We Really Need?

This is obviously an important question and deserves a straightforward answer. To eliminate possible confusion, we need to discuss the Recommended Dietary Allowances (RDAs) because there are RDAs and then there are other RDAs.

RDA can stand for one of two things: recommended *dietary* allowance or recommended *daily* allowance. The way these two terms are usually differentiated is the recommended dietary allowance is abbreviated simply as RDA while the recommended daily allowance is the United States Recommended Daily Allowance, or U.S. RDA.

Recommended dietary allowances were first established in 1943 during World War II after a study by the Food and Nutrition Board of the National Academy of Sciences to determine adequate dietary intakes of essential vitamins and minerals to prevent disease. These recommendations have been updated periodically to reflect our expanding knowledge about disease and nutrition. The last update occurred in 1989. The listing covers 19 different nutrients and makes recommendations for these nutrients based on 18 different age and sex categories. Calcium and vitamin D are two of these nutrients. The actual value of the RDA for each nutrient is the amount that is known to prevent disease, plus an additional amount to provide a margin of safety. Although individual requirements vary, the RDA is calculated to meet the needs of the majority of the population.

U.S. RDAs were established in the 1970s when the Food and Drug Administration (FDA) initiated nutrient labeling on food products. The U.S. RDAs were generally derived from the 1968 edition of the RDAs from the National Academy of Sciences. Their purpose was only to pro-

WOMEN'S AND GIRLS' CALCIUM CONSUMPTION	
Age	Daily Consumption of Calcium in Milligrams
Infant–11	741
12–19	781
20–29	651
30–49	587.5
50–69	575

Source: USDA Nationwide Food Consumption Survey, 1987–1988.

vide consumers with an idea of what percentage of the "real" RDA (the RDA from the National Academy of Science) was contained in an average serving. In other words, the U.S. RDA was intended as a guide to tell how much of a nutrient we were getting, not how much we *should* be getting. Not all nutrients must be listed on food labels. Nutrients that must be listed are protein, vitamin A, vitamin C, thiamine, riboflavin, niacin, calcium, and iron. Vitamin D is considered optional, as are vitamins E, B_6, and B_{12}. When you read a food label, the actual milligrams or grams of the required nutrients are not often listed. Instead, the percentage of the highest 1968 RDA found in the stated serving size is given. For example, on the label of a carton of skim milk you would find a serving size of 1 cup, or 8 ounces. In that 1 serving is 35% of the U.S. RDA for calcium. Unless you know that the U.S. RDA for calcium is 1,000 mg, you have no way of knowing that there are 350 mg of calcium in 1 cup of that brand of skim milk.

In 1990, the United States Congress passed the Nutrition Labeling and Education Act, which set broad standards for food labeling. In response, the FDA developed new regulations, which became effective in May 1994, that changed food labeling requirements. According to the FDA, the changes in labeling reflect most Americans' concerns about getting too much of food components like fat, calories, cholesterol, and sodium. In the case of calcium, however, we are still concerned with getting too little.

The new label for a serving of milk can be compared to the old label most of us grew up with. As you can see, the term U.S. RDA no longer appears. There is a new term called the "% Daily Value." The % Daily Value is the percentage of the recommended amount of the particular nutrient for an individual consuming a 2,000-calorie diet. The actual recommended amounts of the various nutrients for a 2,000-calorie diet and a 2,500-calorie diet are listed at the bottom of the sample label. The nutrients that manufacturers must report in this way include fats, carbohydrates, protein, cholesterol, sodium, and

RDA FOR CALCIUM IN MILLIGRAMS

Age	1963*	1968*	1974	1980	1989
Infants					
0.0–0.5		400/500	360	360	400
0.5–1.0		600	540	540	600
Children					
1–3	800	700/800	800	800	800
4–6	800	800	800	800	800
7–10	800	900/1,000	800	800	800
Males					
11–14	1,100/1,500	1,200/1,400	1,200	1,200	1,200
15–18	1,400	1,400	1,200	1,200	1,200
19–24	800	800	800	800	1,200
25–50	800	800	800	800	800
51+	800	800	800	800	800
Females					
11–14	1,100/1,300	1,200/1,300	1,200	1,200	1,200
15–18	1,300	1,300	1,200	1,200	1,200
19–24	800	800	800	800	1,200
25–50	800	800	800	800	800
51+	800	800	800	800	800
Pregnant	+500	+400	1,200	+400	1,200
Breast feeding					
First 6 months	+500	+500	1,200	+400	1,200
Second 6 months	+500	+500	1,200	+400	1,200

*Some age ranges may have two values because different age ranges were used in these versions of the RDA.

potassium. For vitamins and minerals, like vitamin D and calcium, a new term that describes the recommended amount will also appear. This term replaces the old term "U.S. RDA" and is called the Reference Daily Intake, or RDI. The values for the RDIs for the various vitamins and minerals are exactly the same as the U.S. RDA values. Just as on the old labels, the amount of calcium is reported as a percentage of the Reference Daily Intake or RDI. You will still need to know what the RDI for calcium is to determine the actual milligrams of calcium in a serving. The values for vitamins and minerals used for the U.S. RDAs have not been revised for many years, even though the National Academy of Science RDAs they were based on have undergone multiple revisions. The U.S. RDAs, or what are now called the RDIs, should undergo revisions

soon. They are long overdue. Exactly which values will change, however, remains uncertain.

There is yet another group of "RDAs"! These are the values recommended by the National Institutes of Health's Consensus Development Conference on Optimal Calcium Intake in June 1994. These values were recommended by a panel of experts from all fields of medicine, science, and nutrition. They represent the most comprehensive, common-sense approach to calcium nutrition and osteoporosis.

It's not difficult to understand why the recommended amount of calcium increases as the infant becomes a child and the child becomes an adolescent. The bones of the skeleton are increasing in both length and density during those years. As the rate of growth increases and

---

MILK CARTON LABEL PRIOR TO MAY 1994

LESS THAN 1/2% MILKFAT
PASTEURIZED ◆ GRADE A
NUTRITION INFORMATION PER SERVING

SERVING SIZE ....ONE CUP
SERVINGS PER CONTAINER 8
CALORIES 100

PROTEIN ....10 g	CHOLESTEROL...................5 mg
CARBOHYDRATE...................13 g	SODIUM...................150 mg
FAT...................1 g	POTASSIUM...................340 mg

PERCENTAGE OF U.S. RECOMMENDED DAILY ALLOWANCES
(U.S. RDA)

PROTEIN 25	VITAMIN D 25
VITAMIN A 10	VITAMIN B$_6$ 6
VITAMIN C 6	VITAMIN B$_{12}$ 15
CALCIUM 35	IRON...................0
THIAMINE 8	RIBOFLAVIN 30
NIACIN...................0	MAGNESIUM 10

reaches its peak during adolescence, the amount of calcium necessary to meet the nutritional needs of the body increases. When individuals reach their maximum height and the bones have achieved maximum density or thickness, they need less calcium. As a result, the RDA for calcium is less after the age of 24 than it was between the ages of 10 and 24. The RDA increases during pregnancy and breast feeding because of the infant's demands. But why does the RDA increase for a

---

MILK CARTON LABEL AFTER MAY 1994

NUTRITION FACTS

Serving Size 1 cup
Servings per container 8

Amount Per Serving
Calories 100   Calories from Fat   9

		% Daily Value*
Total Fat	1 g	1.5%
Saturated Fat	0 g	0%
Cholesterol	5 mg	1.7%
Sodium	150 mg	6.3%
Total Carbohydrate	13 g	4.3%
Dietary Fiber	0 g	0%
Sugars	0 g	
Protein	10 g	

Vitamin A 10%		Vitamin C 6%	
Calcium 35%		Iron 0%	
Vitamin D 25%		Vitamin B_6 6%	
Vitamin B_{12} 15%		Thiamine 8%	
Riboflavin 30%		Magnesium 10%	

*Percent Daily Values are based on a 2,000-calorie diet.
Your daily values may be higher or lower, depending on your calorie needs.

	Calories	2,000	2,500
Total Fat	Less than	65 g	80 g
Saturated Fat	Less than	20 g	25 g
Cholesterol	Less than	300 mg	300 mg
Sodium	Less than	2,400 mg	2,400 mg
Total Carbohydrate		300 g	375 g
Fiber		25 g	30 g

Calories per gram:
Fat   9   Carbohydrates   4   Protein   4

NIH's Recommended Levels of Calcium Intake	
Group	**Optimal Daily Intake in Milligrams**
Infants	
Birth–6 months	400
6 months–1 year	600
Children	
1–5 years	800
6–10 years	800–1,200
Adolescents and Young Adults	
11–24 years	1,200–1,500
Men	
25–65 years	1,000
Over 65 years	1,500
Women	
25–50 years	1,000
Over 50 years (postmenopausal)	
On estrogen	1,000
Not on estrogen	1,500
Over 65 years	1,500
Pregnant or Nursing	1,200–1,500

woman after menopause if she does not take estrogen?

In 1978, Drs. Heaney, Recker, and Saville from the Creighton University School of Medicine studied premenopausal women and two groups of postmenopausal women. One group of postmenopausal women was taking estrogen replacement and the other group was not. Using sophisticated methods, the researchers were able to measure not only how much calcium was in the women's customary diet, but how much they actually absorbed from the diet and lost through their urine daily. The premenopausal women and the postmenopausal women who were taking estrogen replacement absorbed calcium from their diets equally well and lost similar amounts of calcium through their urine. In order for these women to meet their bodies' calcium needs while offsetting the losses of calcium in the urine, the doctors calculated that they needed 990 milligrams of calcium a day.

The postmenopausal women not taking estrogen replacement reacted differently. They did not absorb calcium as well as the other two groups and lost more calcium in their urine. Because of the poorer absorption and greater losses of calcium, the doctors calculated that this group of women would need 1,504 mg of calcium every day to stay on an even keel. As an explanation for these findings, they speculated that in some way estrogen actually affected the absorption of calcium from the intestinal tract and the kidneys' ability to conserve calcium. Regardless of the reasons, it became clear that this group of women—women who are postmenopausal and not taking estrogen replacement—needed more calcium. That is why the NOF recommends 1,500 mg of calcium a day for this group.

To find out how much calcium you are getting from your diet now, keep a record of all the food you eat for three to five days and, using any number of commercially available calcium and calorie counters, calculate your average calcium intake per day. It's a good idea to include both weekdays and weekend days. (If you work outside the home Monday through Friday, it's very likely that you eat differently on the weekend.) You need to include days from both time periods to get a truly representative idea of how much calcium you consume. On the other hand, an expedient rule of thumb is that the average American woman's diet, without dairy products, contains about 500 mg of calcium. For each cup of milk you drink, add a round number of 300 mg. For each cup of yogurt, you can add as much as 415 mg (see the appendices). Remember, it's only reasonable to count these things if you consume them every day. If you don't drink at least two 8-ounce glasses of milk every day, or drink a glass of milk and eat a cup of yogurt, it's a safe bet that you are about 500 mg deficient if your RDA is 1,000 mg. If your RDA is 1,500 mg, you are probably 1,000 mg deficient in calcium.

The simple solution to this problem would appear to be regular consumption of dairy products. But they should be low fat; you don't need the milkfat but you do need the calcium. And, as you can see from the list of calcium food values in the appendices, you don't lose any calcium as you go from whole milk down to skim. If adding dairy products to your diet is not possible or if it's simply not for you, there is an alternative: calcium supplements.

CALCIUM SUPPLEMENTS

An enormous number of calcium supplements are available without a prescription. Calcium is actually considered a food additive and not a drug when it is sold as a mineral supplement. This is both good and bad. It means that you do not need a prescription from your doctor in order to purchase it. This helps to keep the cost down and makes it easier to obtain a supplement. It also means that manufacturers of calcium supplements only have to show that their products are safe and that they contain what they say they contain. They do not have to prove to the FDA that their products are effective. As a consequence, there are calcium supplements on the market that, while safe, are not absorbed into your system when you take them. This, of course, makes them worthless.

In choosing a calcium supplement, you should read the label carefully to determine what kind of calcium salt it is, how much elemental calcium is in each tablet, and when the manufacturer recommends you take it.

Refer to the appendices for a list of the many brand-name calcium supplements, categorized by the type of calcium salt they contain. The majority of calcium supplements are calcium carbonate or oyster-shell calcium. Remember, these are identical for all practical purposes. Calcium carbonate is an efficient form of calcium salt. By that, I mean it is possible to get a lot of elemental calcium attached to the carbonate salt. Calcium carbonate is 40% elemental calcium. In 1,000 mg of calcium carbonate, there will be 400 mg of actual calcium. From a practical standpoint, it means that manufacturers can put a lot of calcium into a tablet that is not too big to swallow if they use calcium carbonate. Several different manufacturers make calcium carbonate tablets that contain 500 or 600 mg of elemental calcium. This is often all that is needed to supplement the diet, so only one tablet a day is necessary. That certainly makes things easier.

In contrast, calcium gluconate is only 9% elemental calcium. In 1,000 mg of calcium gluconate, there will be only 90 mg of calcium. You can't find a calcium gluconate supplement that supplies 500 mg of elemental calcium in one tablet, because it would be too large for anyone to swallow.

Some brands have incorporated the amount of elemental calcium into the name of the product. OsCal 500, for example, is a calcium carbonate supplement. Each tablet contains 500 mg of elemental calcium although the amount of calcium carbonate in each tablet is 1,250 mg. Other brands may not indicate the amount

Amounts of Elemental Calcium in Calcium Salts Used as Supplements		
Calcium Salt	Mg of Calcium/ 1,000 mg of Calcium Salt	% Calcium
Calcium Carbonate	400	40.0
Calcium Phosphate Tribasic	388	38.8
Calcium Lactate	184	18.4
Calcium Gluconate	93	9.3
Calcium Citrate	241	24.1

of elemental calcium they contain. Formulations of Citracal, a calcium citrate supplement, have actually used the amount of calcium salt in the name. Citracal 950 was the brand name of a calcium citrate tablet that contained 950 mg of calcium citrate but only 200 mg of elemental calcium. This caused some confusion on the part of consumers who thought that each tablet provided 950 mg of elemental calcium. The company has recently changed the name to just plain Citracal to help avoid confusion. Always read the label to be sure how much elemental calcium you're getting.

The kind of calcium salt also determines when you should take the calcium supplement. Calcium carbonate and calcium phosphate supplements should be taken with food to ensure that they are well absorbed. Calcium citrate should be taken on an empty stomach. (Additional guidelines on when to take the different types of calcium supplements are offered in the appendices.) Some years ago, the recommendation to take calcium supplements at bedtime was widely circulated. There is no overwhelming reason to do this, however, and it's obviously impractical since most supplements should be taken with food.

There are two other good rules of thumb for taking calcium supplements. Never take more than 600 mg of elemental calcium at one time and always drink at least 8 ounces of liquid when swallowing the tablets. Adequate liquid is necessary if the tablet is to dissolve; if the tablet does not dissolve, you can't absorb the calcium. Even if you determine that you need 1,000 mg of elemental calcium to supplement your diet, don't take it all at once. You will need to divide the amount into at least two doses to be sure that you absorb the calcium efficiently.

Never take more than 600 mg of elemental calcium at one time and always drink at least 8 ounces of liquid when swallowing the tablets.

The efficient absorption of calcium from a supplement also depends on the supplement itself. A disturbing report from Drs. C. J. Carr and R. F. Shangraw revealed that many of the calcium supplements being sold in the United States could not pass quality standards established in the United States Pharmacopeia (USP).

The tablets, when tested, did not dissolve or disintegrate within acceptable time limits.

The good news from these studies was that there were well-known commercial brands of calcium supplements that passed these tests. Unfortunately, this information is not always available for the consumer to read on the packaging. Manufacturers do promote these findings in advertisements but these ads are often restricted to medical journals. You should ask your doctor what calcium supplement he or she recommends. You can also call the manufacturer and ask if the product meets USP standards for disintegration and dissolution. If all else fails, there is a test that you can do at home to see if the calcium tablet will disintegrate properly. This is "the vinegar test." Take one calcium tablet and place it in a glass of vinegar at room temperature. Stir vigorously for 30 minutes. At the end of that time, the tablet should have disintegrated into fine particles. If it has not, the tablet is probably not going to disintegrate properly in your stomach.

The vinegar test: take one calcium tablet and place it in a glass of vinegar at room temperature. Stir vigorously for 30 minutes.

Disintegration is not a concern with chewable calcium supplements like TUMS or Supplical. Only tablets that are swallowed must meet disintegration standards. Dissolution is important for all calcium supplements regardless of whether they are chewed or swallowed. Some of the commercially available supplements that have met USP standards are TUMS, Supplical, OsCal 500, and Citracal.

A WORD OF CAUTION

In 1981 there were reports of high levels of lead in dolomite and bone meal, two very inexpensive sources of calcium often used as supplements. Because of this, in the April 1982 FDA Drug Bulletin, physicians were warned to avoid recommending these products for infants, young children, and pregnant or breast-feeding women. In other adults, the lead content was not thought to be dangerous unless individuals took more than two or three times the amounts recommended on the label.

SIDE EFFECTS OF CALCIUM SUPPLEMENTS

Most individuals who take calcium supplements experience no side effects at all. The only two side effects that occur often enough to be called common are constipation and intestinal gas. Constipation can occur because any calcium that is not absorbed may contribute to the development of a hard stool. The key to avoiding constipation is to make absorption maximally effective. Use a supplement that passes USP standards for disintegration and dissolution. Drink a full glass of water or other liquid when taking the supplement. Take the supplement with a meal if directed to do so. And finally, taking smaller doses of calcium several times a day rather than one large dose of calcium improves absorption. These measures should reduce the likelihood of constipation as well as increasing the potential benefit from your calcium supplement.

Intestinal gas is more a function of the type of calcium salt than the calcium itself. Calcium carbonate is the type of calcium salt that reportedly increases gas. Calcium phosphate and calcium citrate are less likely to cause gas, but some of my patients taking these types of supplements have complained of this problem. Chewable calcium tablets may also be more likely to cause gas than tablets that are swallowed. One of the calcium carbonate brands, OsCal, actually has simethicone, which helps to reduce intestinal gas, in its tablet coating. Simethicone is the antigas ingredient commonly found in antacids. Simethicone is not, however, present in the chewable OsCal 500 tablet.

The potential side effect that creates the most concern is the development of kidney stones. Most, but not all, kidney stones contain calcium. It's only reasonable to worry that if you increase the amount of calcium in your diet with either high-calcium foods or calcium supplements, you might increase your risk of developing a kidney stone. People can develop kidney stones even when they consume a very low-calcium diet. Kidney stones can occur because of an infection. They also occur in individuals with structural abnormalities in the kidneys that prevent a normal flow of urine. A functional problem within the kidney itself may allow excessive amounts of calcium to leak into the urine, making a stone more likely to develop. There are also individuals who actually absorb calcium from their diets with a supernormal efficiency. Instead of absorbing only 25% of the calcium they consume, they may absorb 50% to 75%.

Today, when an individual has a kidney stone, the doctor can have the stone analyzed to see if it contains calcium. The doctor can also determine why the stone developed. If an infection is present, it can be treated successfully with antibiotics. Structural abnormalities in the kidneys may require surgery to correct. Improper function of the kidneys that allows leakage of calcium into the urine can generally be corrected with medication. It's important to realize that there are specific causes for kidney stones that can be found and treated. Most of the causes have little or nothing to do with the amount of calcium in the diet. Those individuals who hyperabsorb calcium from their diet do need to avoid high-calcium diets and supplements.

For the individual who is basically healthy, has none of these problems, and has never had a kidney stone before, meeting the appropriate RDA for calcium through the diet or with a supplement is very safe. Exceeding the RDA slightly is also not thought to be harmful, but there is no reason to double or triple the RDA. There is no proof that this is beneficial to the bones and it is possible to overwhelm a healthy kidney with excessive amounts of calcium that could lead to a kidney stone. Kidney stones aren't fatal, but there are very few things that are more painful.

A PLAN

There are two things you must know before proceeding. First, what your RDA is (refer to the NOF chart earlier in this chapter) and, second, how much calcium do you consume in your regular daily diet? If you are meeting your RDA you need not make any changes. If you are not meeting your RDA, you must decide if you can regularly add high-calcium foods (and that really means dairy products) to your diet in sufficient amounts to meet your RDA. If you cannot, then pick a good calcium supplement and take it daily. If you have ever had a kidney stone or been advised by your doctor to avoid dairy products or calcium supplements, check with your doctor and discuss the issue before proceeding. It is never too late to benefit from adequate calcium and, for that matter, it is never too early to begin.

CHAPTER 4

Estrogen's Role in Osteoporosis

In theory, this chapter could be the shortest one in this book. Estrogen replacement at menopause dramatically reduces the risk of developing osteoporosis. Period. This is absolutely certain and not the least bit controversial. If I were to stop right here, you would know one of the most important benefits of estrogen replacement. You would not, however, know all you need to know.

ESTROGEN DEFICIENCY AND OSTEOPOROSIS

Believe it or not, estrogen deficiency was first suggested as a cause of osteoporosis over 50 years ago. Dr. Fuller Albright and two colleagues, Drs. Patricia Smith and Anna Richardson, writing in the *Journal of the American Medical Association* in 1941, described their observations of 42 patients who developed osteoporosis. Forty were postmenopausal women and two were men. Dr. Albright noted that there were no cases of osteoporosis in women before menopause and that estrogen replacement seemed to have a beneficial effect in preventing the disease. In 1941, Drs. Albright, Smith, and Richardson suggested that the "post-menopausal state" was the most common cause of osteoporosis.

Research in this area lagged until the 1970s and 1980s. In 1985, Dr. Bruce Ettinger published the results of a study of postmenopausal women in the *Annals of Internal Medicine*. Dr. Ettinger used hospital records to document the number of fractures that had occurred after menopause in a group of 490 postmenopausal women, half of whom had taken estrogen replacement and half of whom had not. The women were an average age of 73 years old at the time the study was done.

Dr. Ettinger was also able to measure the spine bone density in some, but not all, of the 73-year-old women in the study. Although the average age of the women was 73, the women who had taken estrogen replacement had spinal bone densities that were more characteristic of women who were only 60. The number of fractures that occurred in these two groups was also quite different. Women taking estrogen replacement had 50% fewer fractures than the women who did not take estrogen. This study strongly suggested two important points Fuller Albright had suggested some 40 years earlier: estrogen deficiency plays a part in decreasing bone density and increasing the number of fractures, and estrogen replacement is important in preserving bone density and pre- venting osteoporotic fractures.

Two years later in the *New England Journal of Medicine* information from the famous Framingham Heart

Study* on the use of estrogen replacement and the occurrence of hip fractures was reported. The medical histories of almost 3,000 women were reviewed for the occurrence of hip fracture and estrogen use. Women who had taken postmenopausal estrogen replacement were found to have a 35% lower risk of hip fracture than women who had never taken estrogen replacement.

Estrogen replacement's ability to prevent postmenopausal bone loss was actively being studied even prior to Dr. Ettinger's report. In the *British Medical Journal* in 1973, Dr. Robert Lindsay and his colleagues reported preliminary information from what continues to be one of the most important studies of estrogen replacement today. The women who participated in this research study were all postmenopausal. Some of the women were only 2 months postmenopausal, some were 3 years postmenopausal, and some were 6 years postmenopausal. Most of the women were given estrogen replacement but some of the women were given only a placebo. Bone-density measurements were performed periodically over what was ultimately to be 16 years of study. Several important findings came from this study. The women who were given a placebo steadily lost bone density over the entire 16 years. The women who were given estrogen replacement maintained their bone density throughout the entire 16 years. The women who started estrogen within 2 months of menopause had the greatest bone density, followed by the women who began estrogen 3 years after menopause and then the women who

began estrogen 6 years after menopause. The women who were 3 years postmenopausal when they began estrogen replacement actually demonstrated a slight gain in bone density, although their bone density did not achieve the higher level seen in the women who were only 2 months postmenopausal. The most important conclusion from this study is that estrogen replacement can prevent bone loss at any point in time a postmenopausal woman chooses to take it. The longer a woman waits to begin estrogen replacement, however, the greater the likelihood that she will experience some irreversible bone loss.

The protection from bone loss afforded by estrogen replacement lasts only as long as estrogen replacement is continued. In other words, when estrogen replacement is stopped, bone loss will begin. In a research study in Denmark, women were given estrogen replacement or placebo for 2 years. During that 2-year period, the women in the placebo group steadily lost bone while the women receiving estrogen maintained their bone density. At the end of the 2-year period, some of the women who were given estrogen were changed to a placebo and some of the women who were given a placebo were changed to estrogen. When the women who were on estrogen were given a placebo, they began to lose bone just like the women who had been in the placebo group from the beginning. The women who had been given a placebo initially and were then given estrogen, stopped losing bone immediately.

From the research studies that have been completed to date, we know that

---

*The Framingham Heart Study is a landmark study in which all of the inhabitants of the town of Framingham, Massachusetts, regularly undergo complete medical histories and examinations to document the occurrence of disease. An enormous amount of information about heart disease, high blood pressure, and cholesterol has come from the Framingham Heart Study.

estrogen replacement is effective in stopping bone loss in women up until the age of 80. That doesn't mean that estrogen is ineffective after the age of 80. That just means we don't have sufficient information on women after the age of 80 to say one way or the other.

All of the studies from the medical literature that have documented the ability of estrogen replacement in preventing postmenopausal bone loss and reducing the risk of osteoporotic fractures are too numerous to mention. Suffice it to say that, without question, estrogen replacement can prevent or significantly slow postmenopausal bone loss. With estrogen replacement, the risk of developing osteoporotic fractures is reduced at least 50%.

Why estrogen deficiency causes bone loss remains the subject of today's research. Initially, it was thought that estrogen did not affect the bone directly. Theories were put forth that suggested that in the absence of estrogen, production of other hormones, which were known to affect the bone, was altered and led to bone loss.

In recent years, certain regions of the bone have been identified as sites to which estrogen attaches. These are called estrogen receptors. In fact, these receptors are located on the very cells that are responsible for new bone formation, the osteoblasts. There may be receptors on the cells that cause bone loss, the osteoclasts, as well. We are still not sure exactly what happens when estrogen attaches or "binds" to these receptors. Estrogen may control the production of a group of substances within the bone called cytokines. Many of these substances have been identified in the last few years. Some of these substances appear to cause bone loss and others appear to stimulate new bone formation. In the absence of estrogen, pro-

duction of the cytokines that cause bone loss increases. In the presence of estrogen, production of the cytokines that cause bone formation increases.

The bone loss that occurs at menopause as a result of estrogen deficiency can be rapid. Bone loss in women tends to begin after the age of 30, particularly from the hip. This bone loss occurs because of calcium deficiency, a lack of exercise, smoking, and other largely preventable factors. Nevertheless, it is unfortunately quite common for a woman to begin losing bone after 30. The rate at which she loses bone is about 0.5% to 1% of her bone mass each year. At menopause, when estrogen deficiency becomes profound, the rate of bone loss increases dramatically to between 3% and 7% per year, every year. This rapid bone loss is greatest in the first 3 to 5 years after menopause, but may continue as long as 10 years after the onset of menopause before slowing of its own accord. It is possible then, for a woman to lose 15% to 35% of her bone mass in the first 5 years after menopause without estrogen replacement.

> *It is possible then, for a woman to lose 15% to 35% of her bone mass in the first 5 years after menopause without estrogen replacement.*

WHEN DOES ESTROGEN-DEFICIENT BONE LOSS BEGIN?

That may seem like a strange question. The obvious answer is that estrogen-deficient bone loss begins when we become estrogen deficient. So perhaps the real question is, when do we become estrogen deficient, as least as far as the bones are concerned? A companion question would be, how much estrogen does the bone need to prevent bone loss?

Estrogen levels in the blood begin to decline long before the last menstrual period occurs. To adequately explain this situation, we need to understand what happens in the normal reproductive life of a woman and the changes that take place at menopause.

THE MENSTRUAL CYCLE

Girls usually begin menstruating between the ages of 9 and 16, although the average age is 12. The bleeding generally does not become regular for about a year. Once regular menstrual cycles begin, the levels of estrogen and progesterone rise and fall predictably in the blood. A brief look at the production of hormones by the ovary during a normal menstrual cycle is worthwhile.

When doctors talk about what happens in the menstrual cycle, they number the days of the cycle, calling the first day of menstrual bleeding day 1 of the new cycle. I realize that this is not the way we normally think of the bleeding period. We tend to think the bleeding signals the end of any cycle. Medically speaking, however, day 1 is the first day of the menstrual period. Most menstrual bleeding lasts between 5 and 7 days. During this time, estrogen levels remain low. The estrogen is not gone from the blood, it is just low. At about day 8 or 9 in the cycle, the estrogen levels begin to rise, slowly at first and then much more rapidly, reaching their peak around day 14.

The first 14 days of the menstrual cycle are called the follicular phase. This is because it is during this time that the folli-

cle, which will ultimately release an egg, is developed within the ovary. The follicle is being directed to mature by a hormone made in the pituitary gland called "follicle-stimulating hormone," or FSH. The growing follicle is the source of the estrogen that rises progressively in the blood as the follicle matures. Finally, the follicle is self-sufficient and no longer needs FSH to grow, so FSH production by the pituitary gland drops off. The mature follicle is then ready to release the egg.

The release of the egg, or "ovulation," occurs around day 15. A second hormone from the pituitary gland, called luteinizing hormone, or LH, is suddenly released into the blood by the pituitary gland. This is one of the signals to the ovary to release the egg from the follicle. For the first few days after ovulation, estrogen production by the follicle slows. It gradually picks up again and remains constant until about day 23 when estrogen levels begin to fall. Estrogen levels continue to fall throughout the rest of the 28-day cycle.

Once the follicle releases the egg around day 15, the follicular phase ends and the luteal phase is said to have begun. The follicle is no longer called a follicle. Having released the egg, it now becomes a "corpus luteum." Hence the name luteal phase. The corpus luteum has a reasonably fixed life span of 14 days if pregnancy does not occur. The corpus luteum continues to make estrogen much as it did when it was a developing follicle, but it also now makes a second type of hormone called progesterone.

Progesterone levels in the blood are virtually negligible during the follicular phase of the menstrual cycle. Progesterone is not being produced by the ovary during this time. During the luteal phase, or second half of the cycle, the corpus luteum begins to produce progesterone and maximum levels are reached within 5 days after ovulation, sometime between days 18 and 20. The level of progesterone declines sharply around day 21 or 22 until it reaches its original low level when the next menstrual bleeding begins, which is day 1 of the next menstrual cycle. The level of estrogen also declines sharply around day 21 or 22 and continues to decline until it too reaches its original low level around day 1 of the next menstrual cycle.

Menstrual bleeding occurs because of the fall in the level of estrogen and progesterone. Both of these hormones stimulate the lining of the uterus or womb to grow. This lining is called the endometrium. The purpose of this lining is to provide an area within the uterus for a fertilized egg to develop. If pregnancy does not occur; that is, if the egg is not fertilized by male sperm, the production of estrogen and progesterone diminishes as I described above and the nourishment for the endometrium is withdrawn. As a result, the endometrium is shed in the form of menstrual bleeding.

We talk about the menstrual cycle being 28 days long. However, there are few of us who have menstrual periods exactly every 28 days. What I have described is certainly the textbook version of the normal sequence of events. The follicular phase can be quite variable in its length. If instead of being 14 days long, the follicular phase is 21 days long, the overall menstrual cycle will be 35 days instead of 28. The duration of the luteal phase can change as well, although it is more common for this phase to become shorter, rather than longer. This undoubtedly seems rather complicated. I think that it is important, though, for a woman to understand what is happening to her during the menstrual cycle.

THE MENOPAUSE

Strictly speaking, menopause refers to the last menstrual period that a woman has. Why do we stop menstruating? The simple answer is we run out of eggs.

Before we are born, our ovaries contain several million eggs. By the time we are born, this number has fallen to around 700,000. The eggs have, in essence, died of their own accord. By the time we begin menstruating as teenagers, only about 400,000 eggs remain. Between the time we begin and cease menstruating, we will experience about 400 menstrual cycles. But because the other eggs not involved in the 400 or so menstrual cycles are deteriorating on their own, by the age of 50 there are no more healthy eggs left. Without the production of estrogen and progesterone by the follicle containing the egg, the endometrium does not develop

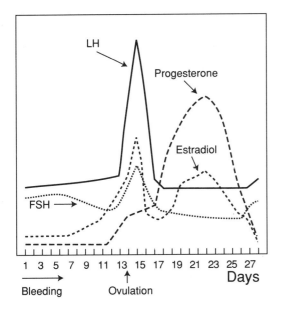

Hormone levels during the cycle.

and so there is no endometrium to bleed during each cycle.

This process does not occur all at once. That is, we do not have perfectly regular cycles for years and then one day abruptly stop. Around the age of 40, it is not uncommon for a woman to begin having irregular cycles. If she usually had a period every 30 days, her periods may begin to occur every 25 days. She may then notice a lengthening of the time between periods to every 40 or 45 days. These changes in the regularity of the periods may be the first signs of approaching menopause.

Another sign is hot flashes, also called flushes, which can occur in women who have not yet reached 40. Hot flashes are just what they sound like. Within a matter of minutes, a woman develops an intense feeling of warmth usually in the face, neck, and chest. She may sense that something is about to happen just before the onset of the hot flash. The feeling of intense warmth usually lasts for 5 or 6 minutes or it may last for an hour. She may perspire heavily during this time, just as she would if she were outside on an especially hot day. There is a marked difference in the way this feels, however, because you are hot from the inside out. It is possible to actually measure a marked increase in the temperature of the skin during a hot flash. The heart also beats faster due to the increased amounts of adrenaline that are released during a hot flash. Once the hot flash subsides, a woman may actually feel quite cold.

These beginning signs of approaching menopause are signals of a decline in the production of estrogen by the ovaries. These symptoms of estrogen deficiency and declining ovarian function have a name all of their own. They are called the climacteric. While the average age of menopause (the last menstrual period) is 50 to 52, the climacteric may span the ages of 35 to 60. The important point here is that even before the ovaries stop producing estrogen completely and the last period occurs, estrogen levels can decline to a level sufficiently low enough to trigger bone loss.

Unfortunately, we don't know exactly what that magic level of estrogen is. We have an idea of what the average level of estrogen is in the blood when bone loss begins, but it is so variable from woman to woman, it is not a useful figure. In other words, we cannot measure your estrogen level and automatically know what your bones might be doing. So what can we do?

HOW TO KNOW IF YOU NEED ESTROGEN REPLACEMENT TO STOP BONE LOSS

Our best and most direct approach is to look at the bones with bone-density testing. This is currently the only reliable means of determining whether a woman needs estrogen replacement to prevent osteoporosis.

Bone-density testing is recommended for women who are approaching menopause. For most women, that means in the late forties. However, if a woman's ovaries are surgically removed before she stops menstruating on her own, she is "surgically menopausal" regardless of her age. Some women become menopausal when they are in their late thirties for reasons we don't understand. So when I say a woman in her late forties should consider bone-density testing, I am referring to the "average" woman who will ultimately become menopausal around the age of 50 to 52.

We have the ability to measure the bone density in many different areas of the skeleton. Almost any area of the skeleton can be measured reasonably well to determine a woman's risk of having a fracture either today or in the future. I prefer to measure the bone in the spine and hips in my patients who are approaching menopause. Spine fractures and hip fractures are the most important types of osteoporotic fracture so I like to measure these areas directly rather than measuring another area and extrapolating that information to the spine and hip. I may also need to look at the spine a year or two after menopause and this first spine measurement serves as a basis for comparison.

The information from the bone density test tells me whether my patient is at any risk of having an osteoporotic fracture now or in the future. This judgement is made based on the bone density that is measured during the test. For example, not too long ago a woman I'll call Sally, who was 45 years old and just beginning to experience some hot flashes and menstrual irregularities, came to see me for an assessment of her risk of developing osteoporosis. A bone-density study of her spine revealed that her bone density was 15% below the average maximum bone density normally seen in a 20-year-old woman. Although this bone density was not low enough to put Sally at risk of having a fracture today, the rate of expected bone loss after menopause would ultimately cause her bone density to fall to that level. As a consequence, I told Sally that she should definitely consider taking estrogen replacement at menopause in order to prevent osteoporosis. In the meantime, of course, I recommended that she meet her recommended daily allowance for calcium and vitamin D and that she exercise regularly.

Another woman, whom I will call Helen, came to see me for similar reasons. Helen was also in her late forties and beginning to have some menstrual irregularities, but unlike Sally, when we measured the bone density in her spine her bone density was already so low that she was at risk for osteoporotic fractures now. Helen was otherwise quite healthy. I could not determine any medical reason for Helen having such a low bone density. Helen's low bone density probably represented a very low peak bone density. The fact remained that Helen could ill afford any bone loss at all. I recommended that we start estrogen replacement immediately rather than waiting for her periods to completely stop on their own. I did not want her to risk even brief periods of estrogen deficiency, which could cause bone loss.

Barbara's concerns were somewhat different when I saw her. Her periods had stopped about 6 months before our visit, but she felt well. She was not having hot flashes and did not wish to take estrogen replacement unless she clearly needed it. She realized, however, that she had no way of knowing what was happening to her bones. She came to see me to ask for my advice. Barbara is a very slender, petite woman. Her small size would tend to make you think that she might be a woman who will develop osteoporosis. However, when I measured her spine and hip bone density, I found that Barbara, at the age of 55, still had bone densities in the spine and hip that were actually 14% better than what we consider to be the average maximum bone density of a 20-year-old woman! Why were her bones so good? Part of the reason is almost certainly her inheritance. That is, she inherited the ability to make a greater amount of bone than average. She also had always exercised regularly, met her RDA for calcium, and had never smoked. With her superb bone densities at the age of 55, it was highly unlikely that Barbara would ever develop osteoporosis, even without estrogen replacement. I could tell Barbara that it was not necessary for her to begin estrogen replacement to prevent osteoporosis. I did tell her to keep taking her calcium supplement and to continue exercising.

Women certainly take estrogen replacement at menopause for other reasons besides preventing osteoporosis. Distressing hot flashes can be relieved with estrogen. Drying and thinning of the vaginal lining, which can lead to recurrent infections and painful intercourse, can be prevented or treated with estrogen. Some women simply report that their overall well-being is dependent on taking estrogen replacement. There is also accumulating evidence that estrogen may play a role in the prevention of heart disease. For a more extensive discussion of the issues surrounding estrogen replacement and menopause, I encourage you to read Dr. Lila Nachtigall's book, *Estrogen: The Facts that Can Change Your Life!,* and Dr. Wulf Utian's book, *Managing Your Menopause.* (See the appendices for more information on these and other books on menopause.)

Even if you begin estrogen replacement for reasons that have nothing to do with the prevention of osteoporosis, before you stop estrogen-replacement therapy, or ERT, you must consider what may happen to your bones without estrogen. For example, a woman may begin estrogen replacement to stop hot flashes. After 4 or 5 years she may wish to try to stop estrogen replacement with the expectation that the hot flashes will not return. But what about her bones? If she has never had a bone-density test done, she cannot know whether she might be at risk for osteoporosis if she stops her estrogen replacement. So, even if a woman begins estrogen

for reasons other than the prevention of osteoporosis, I encourage her to have a bone-density test done before stopping estrogen.

FDA-APPROVED ESTROGENS FOR THE PREVENTION OF OSTEOPOROSIS

At the present time, four estrogen products have been approved by the FDA for the prevention of osteoporosis. In the future, there undoubtedly will be more. There are certainly more than four estrogen preparations that are available by prescription for menopausal women for estrogen replacement. We have no reason to believe that the other types of estrogen replacement are ineffective in preventing osteoporosis, but the research that would prove otherwise has not yet been done. We also haven't identified the exact dose of estrogen these other preparations must contain to protect the bones. Some of the doses we might use for hot flashes or vaginal dryness, for example, may not be enough to protect the bones.

Doctors may prescribe different forms of estrogens for a menopausal woman. By that I mean there are estrogen pills, injections, vaginal creams, topical gels, estrogen pellets, and an estrogen patch. Estrogen gels, which are applied to the skin, are not approved for use in the United States. Similarly, estrogen pellets that release estrogen slowly and are surgically implanted under the skin are also not approved for use in the United States. Vaginal estrogen products are intended to relieve vaginal dryness and irritation that comes from estrogen deficiency. Estrogen does reach the bloodstream when these preparations are used, but the amount that enters the blood can be so erratic that we cannot use vaginal creams to prevent osteoporosis. Three estrogen pill formulations and one estrogen patch have been approved by the FDA for the prevention of osteoporosis. They are Premarin, Estrace, Ogen, and Estraderm™, respectively.

PREMARIN (CONJUGATED EQUINE ESTROGEN)

Premarin was the first form of estrogen replacement approved by the FDA for the prevention of osteoporosis. (It is made by Wyeth-Ayerst Pharmaceuticals in Philadelphia, Pennsylvania.) For many years, Premarin has been the mainstay of estrogen replacement for menopausal women. A Premarin tablet has a characteristic football shape, a slick coating, and cannot be easily broken or halved. Five different strengths are available and are identifiable by their color. The green is a 0.3 mg tablet, the burgundy is 0.625 mg, the white is 0.9

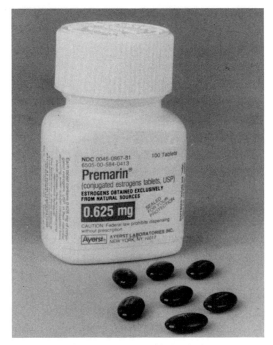

Premarin. Photo courtesy of Wyeth-Ayerst Laboratories, Philadelphia, Pennsylvania. The appearance of these tablets is a trademark of Wyeth-Ayerst Laboratories.

mg, the yellow is 1.25 mg, and the violet is 2.5 mg. The major type of estrogen found in Premarin is called estrone. Estrone and estradiol are the two major types of estrogen normally made by a woman's ovaries. Estradiol is actually the more potent and important type of estrogen. The body, however, can take estrone and convert it to estradiol rapidly. Indeed, this is what happens when you take Premarin.

Premarin also contains equilin estrogens. These are estrogens that are normally found in horses but that are active in human beings as well. While that may sound strange, I assure you Premarin has been used for many years quite safely and effectively. In medical studies that have looked at the ability of Premarin to stop bone loss due to estrogen deficiency, the smallest dose that appeared to be effective was the burgundy 0.625 mg tablet. We therefore say that, in general, the "minimum effective dose" of Premarin is 0.625 mg. An individual woman might need more than that or she might need less. The dose of 0.625 mg is considered the "starting" dose when Premarin is prescribed to prevent osteoporosis.

OGEN (ESTROPIPATE)

Ogen is also an oral form of estrogen replacement. By oral form, I mean that it is available as a pill or tablet. Like Premarin, the type of estrogen in Ogen is estrone.

Ogen does not, however, contain equilin estrogens. The Ogen tablet is oblong in shape and is scored so that the tablet can be cut in half if necessary. Four different tablet strengths of Ogen, which are also identifiable by color, are available. The Ogen 0.625-mg tablet is pale yellow, the 1.25-mg tablet is peach, the 2.5-mg tablet is light blue, and the 5-mg tablet is pale green. Although some of these tablet

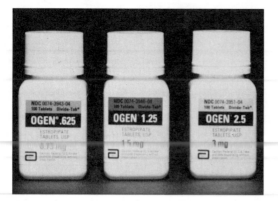

Ogen. Photo courtesy of Abbott Laboratories, Abbott Park, Illinois.

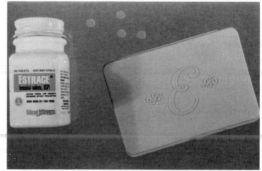

Estrace, oral 17-B estradiol. Manufactured by Bristol-Myers Squibb Co.

strengths are similar to those available for Premarin, the absence of the equilin estrogens in Ogen makes it a bit less potent, milligram for milligram, than Premarin. But in research studies, like Premarin, the minimum effective dose of Ogen was the 0.625-mg dose.

ESTRACE (MICRONIZED ESTRADIOL)

Estrace is an estrogen tablet that contains the more potent estradiol instead of estrone. However, the type of estrogen that circulates in the blood is primarily estrone. In the intestinal tract and liver, the estradiol in Estrace is rapidly converted to estrone. Remember, the body can convert estrone back to estradiol and estradiol to estrone. Because Estrace is originally estradiol, blood levels of estradiol reach slightly higher levels with Estrace than with Premarin or Ogen. There are three strengths of Estrace available, and the small, round tablets are scored so that they can be cut in half easily. The 0.5 mg Estrace tablet is white, the 1 mg tablet is lavender, and the 2 mg tablet is turquoise. Research studies using Estrace have

demonstrated that the smallest dose of Estrace that will prevent bone loss is 0.5 mg, or one-half of the 1-mg tablet.

ESTRADERM™ (ESTRADIOL TRANSDERMAL SYSTEM)

Ciba Pharmaceutical Company makes Estraderm™ (estradiol transdermal system). The form of estrogen contained in Estraderm™ (estradiol transdermal system) is estradiol. This is not an estrogen pill; the estradiol is incorporated into a patch that is worn on the abdomen or hip. When placed on the skin, estradiol is released through what is called the control membrane. The skin itself also controls the amount of estradiol entering the body. The estradiol is then picked up by the blood and enters the general circulation. Some of this estradiol will be converted to estrone, but the type of estrogen that circulates in the blood remains predominantly estradiol. There are only two strengths of the Estraderm patch available at present. The 0.05-mg patch is about the size of a silver dollar. The 0.1-mg patch is more oblong in shape and is about 3 inches long. The patch is placed on the abdomen or hip and worn for 3½ days. A new patch is then applied to another area of the abdomen or hip. You can bath, shower, or swim while wearing the patch. The adhesive that holds the patch in place is waterproof. (Some women have reported skin irritation from the adhesive although this is usually mild.)

In studies using different strengths of Estraderm™ (estradiol transdermal system) to prevent bone loss, the 0.05-mg patch was found to be the lowest dose that was effective in protecting the bone mass.

WHICH KIND OF ESTROGEN SHOULD YOU TAKE TO PREVENT OSTEOPOROSIS?

All four of these forms of estrogen replacement have been proven to be effective in preventing bone loss *as long as the correct dose is given.* Although we know what the minimum effective doses of these four forms are, this does not mean that they are the correct doses for *every* woman. This does mean that doses smaller than these have generally been found to be ineffective in preventing bone loss.

The decision regarding which estrogen to use is not based on the prevention of osteoporosis because all of these estrogens are effective in that regard. The choice is between taking a pill or wearing a patch, which is simply a matter of personal preference. The tablets are taken every day and the patch is changed twice a week.

Medically speaking, there are differences between taking estrogen in pill form and receiving estrogen through the skin from the patch. The most important difference appears to be that oral estrogens, once they are absorbed into the bloodstream, are immediately sent through the circulation in the liver. As a consequence, a large amount of estrogen circulates through the liver. Estrogen delivered from the patch enters the general circulation first, so only a small amount of estrogen is ultimately circulated through the liver at any one time.

The circulation of a lot of estrogen through the liver can, in theory, be both good and bad. One of the good effects of estrogen circulating through the liver is that total cholesterol levels decrease and the good cholesterol level, the HDL level, tends to increase. This should have a beneficial effect on the risk of heart disease. The patch also has a beneficial effect on cholesterol, but it is not as dramatic as the effect of the oral estrogens. Scientists

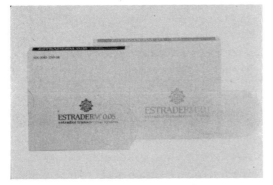

Estraderm™ (estradiol transdermal system). Estraderm™ is a registered trademark of Ciba-Geigy Corporation.

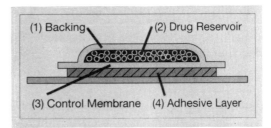

Estraderm™ (estradiol transdermal system). © 1993, Ciba-Geigy Corporation.

MINIMUM EFFECTIVE DOSES OF FDA-APPROVED ESTROGENS FOR THE PREVENTION OF OSTEOPOROSIS	
Type of Estrogen	Minimum Effective Dose
Premarin	0.625 mg
Ogen	0.625 mg
Estrace	0.5 mg
Estraderm™ (estradiol transdermal system) patch	0.05 mg

speculate, however, that estrogen may act on the blood vessels directly to help prevent heart disease. If that is so, it may not matter how estrogen is delivered to the bloodstream or what route it takes. If your cholesterol levels are low to begin with, you may not need the cholesterol-lowering effect of the oral estrogens.

Smoking is known to interact with estrogen in the liver, rendering the estrogen less effective. In a woman who smokes, the use of an estrogen preparation like the patch, in which large amounts of estrogen do not circulate through the liver, would seem to be preferable. The best course of action would be, of course, to stop smoking.

The other consequences (such as high blood pressure and gallstones) of estrogen circulating through the liver in large amounts may be more theoretical than real. These are issues you should thoroughly discuss with your doctor. The most important point to keep in mind is that all of these estrogens are effective in preventing osteoporosis. After that, it is simply a matter of picking the one that is right for you.

DOES ESTROGEN REPLACEMENT CAUSE CANCER?

The very question understandably causes considerable fear in the hearts of many women. Unfortunately, there are women who would benefit from estrogen replacement who deny themselves that benefit because the question, *not the answer,* causes so much fear.

Endometrial cancer is clearly linked to postmenopausal estrogen replacement. Speculation that estrogen could cause this cancer of the uterus' lining followed the observation that women who had tumors that produced excessive amounts of estrogen often developed endometrial cancer as well. In the mid-1970s, there were several reports in the medical literature of increasing numbers of postmenopausal women who were using estrogen replacement and developed endometrial cancer.

Although endometrial cancer is predominantly a disease of postmenopausal women, about 5% of the cases occur in premenopausal women. Interestingly, these women often had recurrent, anovulatory menstrual cycles. In other words, they did not ovulate. Because they did not ovulate, the follicle within the ovary did not become a corpus luteum. That means that no progesterone was produced. This was interesting because researchers realized that the majority of endometrial cancer cases in postmenopausal women taking estrogen were in women who were taking estrogen alone. They were not taking the second hormone progesterone. So, depending upon your perspective, it was not the presence of estrogen that caused the endometrial cancer. It was the absence of progesterone.

A host of studies in the mid- to late 1970s reported that the use of "unopposed estrogen" (the phrase used to describe prescribing estrogen replacement alone without progesterone) could result in as much as a 20-fold increase in a woman's risk of developing endometrial cancer. Most authorities now believe that the longer a woman takes unopposed estrogen replacement, the greater is her risk of developing endometrial cancer. With unopposed estrogen use for 10 to 20 years, the risk increases 8-fold.

The obvious solution to this problem was not to stop prescribing estrogen but rather to add progesterone to the hormone replacement regimen of postmenopausal women. This approach was actually pioneered at Wilford Hall United States Air Force Medical Center in 1971. The first attempts at this type of hormone replacement involved adding progesterone for 5 to 7 days each calendar month. After several years of study, it became clear that this length of time was insufficient to prevent the development of the precancerous state called endometrial hyperplasia. Doctors at Wilford Hall as well as elsewhere concluded that at least 13 days of progesterone were necessary to prevent the development of hyperplasia. This is not terribly surprising when you think about it. After all, under normal circumstances in the luteal phase of the menstrual cycle the ovaries produce progesterone for about 14 days.

The addition of progesterone in this cyclic fashion, 13 days each calendar month, clearly made a difference in the occurrence of endometrial cancer in postmenopausal women taking estrogen. In the Wilford Hall study, endometrial cancer developed in 359 out of every 100,000 women who took estrogen alone. In the women who took both estrogen and progesterone, cancer developed in only 56 out of every 100,000. The result in the estrogen-progesterone group was actually better than the result in postmenopausal women who took no hormones at all. In

fact, a woman who takes at least 10 days of progesterone in addition to estrogen replacement after menopause is estimated to have a 10% lower risk of endometrial cancer than a woman who does not take any hormones at all.

A woman who takes at least 10 days of progesterone in addition to estrogen replacement after menopause is estimated to have a 10% lower risk of endometrial cancer than a woman who does not take any hormones at all.

When progesterone is added in a cyclic fashion to a woman's estrogen-replacement regimen, the progesterone essentially turns off the biochemical machinery within the endometrium that has been set in motion by the estrogen. When the progesterone is stopped after 13 days, the endometrium is shed. Shedding occurs in the form of menstrual bleeding. For most postmenopausal women, this bleeding is generally lighter and shorter in duration than what they experienced premenopausally. The need to prevent endometrial cancer has created something of a trade-off. In order to benefit from estrogen replacement without incurring the risk of endometrial cancer, we have had to accept the indefinite continuation of menstrual periods.

Progesterone is available by prescription. For many years, no medication duplicated the body's natural progesterone exactly. Instead, we used a group of medications called progestins. These are synthetic compounds that are similar to progesterone in their actions. Both progesterone and progestins can be used effectively to prevent endometrial cancer as part of a postmenopausal woman's hormone-replacement regimen. In 1972, only about 10% of women who were prescribed estrogen replacement were also prescribed a progestin. By 1983, that number had risen to 98.7%—and with good reason.

Fortunately, endometrial cancer, when it does occur, has one of the highest cure rates of any type of cancer. The 5-year survival rate is generally reported to be over 90%.

Breast cancer is a much more difficult issue. Our fear of this cancer is greater because the consequences are more serious and we lack the knowledge to answer the most important questions. The problem is *not* that we know that estrogen causes breast cancer. The problem is that we don't know what *does* cause breast cancer.

The hormone estrogen has always been a suspect in this disease. Clearly the breasts are an estrogen-sensitive tissue. Observations of large populations of women had suggested that the younger a woman was when she began menstruating (and therefore producing more estrogen) the more likely she was to develop breast cancer. On the other hand, women who became menopausal prematurely (and therefore lost their estrogen production sooner) seemed to have less risk of developing breast cancer. It was also noted that, in general, the greatest increase in the number of breast cancer cases occurred before menopause. After menopause, fewer new cases of breast cancer were seen. Although the best attorney would agree that this evidence is circumstantial and does not prove that estrogen causes breast cancer, it is sufficient evidence to bring the case to trial. Sadly, this case has been in court for over 2 decades and we still haven't reached a verdict despite very close examination of the facts.

In estrogen's defense, breast cancer does occur in postmenopausal women who have never taken estrogen replacement. In addition, there are some types of breast cancer that, under the microscope, do not have the sites called estrogen receptors required for estrogen action on the cancer cell. In addition, in studies that have looked at the number of deaths that occur in women who develop breast cancer while taking estrogen replacement as compared with those who develop breast cancer and were not taking estrogen, the death rate has been found to be lower in women on estrogen replacement. And finally, there are some types of breast cancer that actually respond to treatment with high doses of synthetic estrogen.

Medical science has been unable to resolve these issues at present. As women, we all have a terrible risk of breast cancer. One out of every nine women may develop breast cancer in her lifetime. Certainly, we do not want to increase that risk. The question we must address is not "What causes breast cancer in the first place?," but "Will postmenopausal estrogen replacement increase the risk of breast cancer that we as women already have?"

In the last several years, there have been extensive attempts to review and combine all of the information ever reported on the development of breast cancer in postmenopausal women taking estrogen replacement. Researchers refer to this as "meta-analysis" of the medical literature. In January 1991, one such meta-analysis concluded that postmenopausal hormone replacement that used a dose of 0.625 mg of conjugated equine estrogen or its equivalent did not cause an increase in breast cancer risk. A second meta-analysis published in the spring of 1991 concluded that there was no increased risk of breast cancer for the first 5 years of use of estrogen replacement but after 15 years of use, a woman's risk of breast cancer was increased by 30%. In 1992, the American College of Physicians published its own meta-analysis of all the studies published since 1970. After a careful review, the College concluded that they could not prove that there was any increase in the risk of breast cancer for women who had used estrogen replacement for five years or less. With longer estrogen use ranging from 10 to 20 years, a woman's risk of breast cancer increased by 25%. To understand what this means, think about it this way: if your risk of breast cancer were doubled, your risk would increase 100%.

Finally, Dr. Janet Henrich, at the Yale University School of Medicine, reviewed the meta-analyses that had been done as well as 24 individual studies of postmenopausal hormone use and breast cancer. This article was published in the *Journal of the American Medical Association* in October of 1992. Dr. Henrich concluded that none of the studies proved an overall increased risk of breast cancer from postmenopausal estrogen use. She also concluded that increased breast cancer risk for long-term estrogen use was also not conclusively proven.

What does this mean for you and me as women? It means that because we have a terrible risk of breast cancer, we must follow our physicians' recommendations for mammography. We also need to learn how to properly perform breast self-examination. Until we learn what causes a normal breast cell to become cancerous, early detection of breast cancer by self-examination and mammography is our best protection. We must also keep an appropriate perspective and not allow our fears to prevent us from benefitting from

what we know. For the average woman, the risk of developing osteoporosis is greater than her risk of developing breast and endometrial cancer combined.

For the average woman, the risk of developing osteoporosis is greater than her risk of developing breast and endometrial cancer combined.

POSTMENOPAUSAL HORMONE-REPLACEMENT REGIMENS

The guiding consideration in choosing an estrogen-replacement regimen is a woman's risk of developing endometrial cancer. If you have had a hysterectomy, which is the surgical removal of the uterus or womb, you cannot develop endometrial cancer. This greatly simplifies the choice of an estrogen-replacement regimen. You can take estrogen replacement daily, without interruption and without fear of endometrial cancer or intermittent bleeding. In general, the second hormone, progesterone or a progestin, would not be prescribed for you. (At present, the only compelling reason to add a progestin or progesterone to an estrogen-replacement regimen is to prevent endometrial cancer, which is not a concern in this instance.)

If you have not had a hysterectomy, the choices are more complex. As I noted earlier, if you are given estrogen alone (it doesn't matter what kind) your risk of developing endometrial cancer will increase. To counteract this increased risk, it is customary to add the second hormone, progesterone or a progestin, to the estrogen-replacement regimen. When both hormones are used in a postmenopausal woman, doctors refer to this as hormone replacement therapy, or HRT, instead of just estrogen-replacement therapy, or ERT.

For many years, doctors used a hormone-replacement regimen in which a woman took estrogen replacement for the first 21 or 25 days of each calendar month. For the last 10 days that she took her estrogen, she also took a tablet that contained a progestin or progesterone. Then, both hormones were stopped for the remainder of the month. Between 36 and 48 hours after stopping both hormones, bleeding similar to that experienced during a menstrual period would be expected to begin. On the first day of the following month, a woman would again begin taking her estrogen replacement.

This regimen has been our old reliable or standard approach to HRT for many years. It served its purpose reasonably well. It delivered the estrogen women needed and the progesterone needed to prevent endometrial cancer. Unfortunately, it did not provide the best quality of life for postmenopausal women. As a consequence, many women totally abandoned hormone replacement, losing the benefits of estrogen replacement. Why?

Depending upon the number of days in the calendar month, a woman who stopped her estrogen after day 21 was estrogen deficient for 7 to 10 days. If she stopped her estrogen on day 25, she was estrogen deficient for 3 to 7 days. During this period of time, symptoms of estrogen deficiency would begin to appear. Hot flashes, fatigue, irritability, and difficulty sleeping could contribute to a poor quality of life during this time. It is also reasonable to assume that some bone loss could occur during this period as well. In looking at the reasons why doctors asked a woman to stop her estrogen replacement for several days each month, it became apparent that

the reasons really weren't very sound. For example, it is not necessary to stop the estrogen in order to protect a woman from endometrial cancer. The progesterone would do that. The bleeding will occur after the progesterone is stopped regardless of whether the estrogen is continued. There is no evidence that stopping the estrogen has any effect on the risk of breast cancer. While it is reasonable to stop the estrogen for a few days if the breasts become tender, there is no reason to stop it routinely in the absence of breast tenderness. The only thing we really accomplished by stopping the estrogen was to make some women feel miserable for several days each month. So the first change to the old regimen was to have women use estrogen replacement on a daily basis, without stopping it at any time during the month.

The use of a progestin remains a necessity if we are to reduce the risk of endometrial cancer in a woman who takes estrogen and has not had a hysterectomy. In recent years, we have learned that the number of days a woman takes the progestin is more important in accomplishing this than the daily dose of the progestin. This is important, because as we lower the dose of the progestin, we also lower the potential for unpleasant side effects from the progestin like bloating, fluid retention, headaches, and breast tenderness. Much smaller doses of progestin are being used now than even 5 years ago. The ideal length of time to take the progestin appears to be 13 days. It doesn't matter whether it is the first 13 days of the month or the last 13 days. This actually allows you to pick when the bleeding will occur. Frankly, it may be easier to remember to take the progestin by the calendar, taking it from the first of the month to the 13th, rather than the 15th through the 28th. This also means that bleeding would occur

TRADITIONAL HRT SCHEDULE							
Mon.	Tues.	Wed.	Thurs.	Fri.	Sat.	Sun.
	1 E	2 E	3 E	4 E	5 E	6 E
7 E	8 E	9 E	10 E	11 E	12 E	13 E
14 E	15 E + P	16 E + P	17 E + P	18 E + P	19 E + P	20 E + P
21 E + P	22 E + P	23 E + P	24 E + P	25 E + P	26 N	27 N
28 N	29 N	30 N	This is how a woman would take estrogen and a progestin when following the traditional hormone-replacement regimen. E = Estrogen. P = Progesterone. N = No hormones. Bleeding is expected to occur on this regimen around day 26 or 27.			

in the middle of the month rather than at the end. You can choose whatever suits your lifestyle best.

The use of daily estrogen, the reduction in the doses of progestins and the flexibility of choosing when bleeding occurs have greatly improved the standard hormone-replacement regimen. The fact remains though, that monthly bleeding is expected from this regimen. While most women accept the monthly occurrence of bleeding as a fact of life, it is also something that most look forward to stopping at menopause. What we would really like to do is to be able to take the estrogen we need, not increase the risk of endometrial cancer, and avoid the indefinite continuation of monthly bleeding. This is the rationale behind the newest hormone-replacement regimen, which is often called the continuous-combined regimen.

In this regimen, estrogen replacement is again used daily. Unlike the standard hormone-replacement regimen in which the progestin or progesterone is taken for 13 days of each calendar month,

in the continuous-combined regimen, a very small dose of the progestin is also taken daily. For the first 6 months that a woman uses this regimen, she may (and almost always does) have some unpredictable bleeding. After the first 6 months she may have no bleeding at all—ever again. The combined, continuous use of the estrogen and progestin finally makes the endometrium unresponsive to the hormones. We think that this will prevent the development of endometrial cancer. In one study that involved over 1,300 women, 1% or less of the women using the continuous-combined hormone-replacement therapy developed the precancerous condition called endometrial hyperplasia after one year. Although the success rate is not 100% in stopping bleeding even after 6 months of combined hormone use, about 61% of women who use this regimen have no bleeding by the end of one year of using this regimen.

One other regimen is being evaluated for use in postmenopausal hormone replacement. Just as in the standard and

ONE SCHEDULE FOR THE NEW STANDARD CYCLIC HORMONE-REPLACEMENT REGIMEN						
Mon.	Tues.	Wed.	Thurs.	Fri.	Sat.	Sun.
	1 E	2 E	3 E	4 E	5 E	6 E
7 E	8 E	9 E	10 E	11 E	12 E	13 E
14 E	15 E	16 E	17 E	18 E + P	19 E + P	20 E + P
21 E + P	22 E + P	23 E + P	24 E + P	25 E + P	26 E + P	27 E + P
28 E + P	29 E + P	30 E + P	E = Estrogen. P = Progesterone. Bleeding will occur around day 1 or 2 of the following month.			

ANOTHER SCHEDULE FOR THE NEW STANDARD CYCLIC HORMONE-REPLACEMENT REGIMEN						
Mon.	Tues.	Wed.	Thurs.	Fri.	Sat.	Sun.
	1 E + P	2 E + P	3 E + P	4 E + P	5 E + P	6 E + P
7 E + P	8 E + P	9 E + P	10 E + P	11 E + P	12 E + P	13 E + P
14 E	15 E	16 E	17 E	18 E	19 E	20 E
21 E	22 E	23 E	24 E	25 E	26 E	27 E
28 E	29 E	30 E	E = Estrogen. P = Progesterone. Bleeding would be expected to occur around day 14 or 15.			

continuous-combined regimens, estrogen is taken daily. The progestin, however, is taken in standard doses for 13 days only once every 3 months. This means that bleeding will occur only once every three months. This is obviously a compromise regimen. A woman takes the progestin only once every 3 months and bleeding, while it still does occur, only occurs once every 3 months. Early reports suggest that this regimen will prevent endometrial cancer, but it is still too early to be sure.

Of course, all of these regimens that combine estrogen and a progestin in any fashion mean that you must take two pills or wear a patch and take a pill. It

SCHEDULE FOR THE CONTINUOUS-COMBINED REGIMEN						
Mon.	Tues.	Wed.	Thurs.	Fri.	Sat.	Sun.
	1	2	3	4	5	6
	E + P	E + P	E + P	E + P	E + P	E + P
7	8	9	10	11	12	13
E + P	E + P	E + P	E + P	E + P	E + P	E + P
14	15	16	17	18	19	20
E + P	E + P	E + P	E + P	E + P	E + P	E + P
21	22	23	24	25	26	27
E + P	E + P	E + P	E + P	E + P	E + P	E + P
28	29	30	E = Estrogen. P = Progesterone. Bleeding is not supposed to occur after six months of therapy on this regimen.			
E + P	E + P	E + P				

means two prescriptions from your physician and two drugs to buy. There are two new products on the market that attempt to make life a little easier. Both contain Premarin, which is FDA-approved for the prevention and treatment of osteoporosis. PremPhase is intended to be used by the woman who is taking estrogen and progestin in the standard cyclic hormone-replacement regimen. PremPro can be used by the woman taking estrogen and progestin in the continuous-combined hormone-replacement regimen. The tablets for both of these products come in blister packs in which you punch the tablet out of the card. The tablets are conveniently arranged in rows on the card with each row providing tablets for one week. For PremPhase, the first two rows of 7 tablets each contain Premarin 0.625 mg only. The last two rows contain a combination of the same dose of Premarin and 5 mg of the progestin called Cycrin, which is a brand of medroxyprogesterone acetate. This eliminates the need to take two pills during the last half of the monthly cycle. The

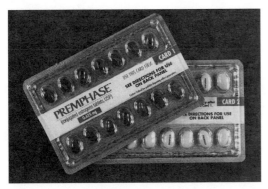

PremPhase. *The appearance of these tablets is a registered trademark of Wyeth-Ayerst.* Photo courtesy of D. McBee, Media Services, Texas Woman's University, Denton, Texas.

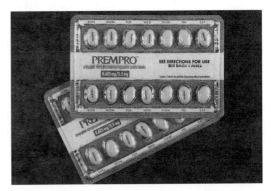

PremPro. *The appearance of these tablets is a registered trademark of Wyeth-Ayerst.* Photo courtesy of D. McBee, Media Services, Texas Woman's University, Denton, Texas.

PremPro tablets all contain Premarin in a dose of 0.625 mg and Cycrin in a dose of 2.5 mg. These peach-colored tablets are taken every day throughout the cycle, again eliminating the need to take two tablets. If a woman uses the Estraderm patch, she must still take a tablet form of a progestin to protect herself from endometrial cancer. A combination estrogen-progesterone patch is being tested in research, so perhaps we will have this desirable option available to use in the near future.

WHEN YOU REACH MENOPAUSE . . .

The most important thing you should do is to discuss your potential need for estrogen replacement with your physician. Even if you feel entirely well without estrogen replacement, remember you cannot know what is happening to your bones. If you have doubts about taking estrogen replacement, a bone-density test can tell you if you are at risk for osteoporosis.

Hormone-replacement regimens are improving. We now have a variety of estrogens to choose from and regimens that recognize that our quality of life is important. Most of the side effects from estrogen or progestin that have troubled women in the past can now be avoided or minimized by carefully selecting the type and dose of the hormones used and the regimen. As my colleague Dr. Lila Nachtigall, professor of obstetrics and gynecology at New York School of Medicine, repeatedly teaches doctors in her lectures, with just a little work, we can get our hormone-replacement regimens right for every woman who needs them. As women, we shouldn't settle for anything less.

CHAPTER 5

Another Look at Smoking and Caffeine

———

Volumes have been written on the ills of smoking, such as emphysema, bronchitis, lung cancer, and heart disease. You really shouldn't need one more reason not to smoke. But just in case you do, smoking increases your risk of osteoporosis. Not only does it increase your risk of osteoporosis, smoking robs you of the very hormones that are so important to women: our estrogens.

Smoking has long been associated with an increased risk of osteoporosis. The question was, how could smoking affect the bones? Did something in the cigarette smoke, like nicotine or carbon monoxide, work directly on the bone to poison it? Could smoking cause a decrease in the amount of estrogen the ovaries made? Could smoking poison the ovaries directly? Or could smoking in some way cause the estrogen made by the ovaries to become ineffective? The evidence suggests that smoking poisons the ovaries and renders the estrogens they produce less effective.

NORMAL ESTROGEN METABOLISM

The female reproductive organs, the ovaries, normally produce two major types of estrogen: estradiol and estrone. Both of these hormones are active in the body. Estradiol is the more potent and abundant of the two hormones. After these hormones are produced in the ovaries, they are released into the circulation where they ultimately make their way to the liver. Within the liver, these estrogens undergo chemical changes, some of which lead to the elimination of estrogen from the body through the kidneys. Another way of saying this is that estrogens undergo hepatic (liver) metabolism.

In the liver, estradiol is changed into estrone and estrone can be changed into estradiol. The whole process can be reversed if the body deems it necessary to maintain the correct level of hormones within the system. The liver can also take estrone and turn it into a third type of estrogen called estriol. This third estrogen causes effects within the body like the other estrogens, estradiol and estrone, but it is much less potent.

The liver can also take estrone and change it into a form of estrogen called 2-hydroxy-estrone. This form of estrogen has no activity in the body and is rapidly taken out of the circulation. It's worthless, as estrogen goes. This form of estrogen cannot protect the bones from bone loss. Once estrone becomes 2-hydroxy-estrone, it cannot be changed back into estrone or estradiol.

THE EFFECTS OF SMOKING ON ESTROGEN METABOLISM

In 1986, the *New England Journal of Medicine* reported that smoking increased the conversion of estrone into the relatively worthless 2-hydroxy-estrone. This reduced the amount of estrone available for conversion back to estradiol or for conversion to estriol. This study was done with premenopausal women who smoked at least 15 cigarettes per day.

There has also been speculation that the amount of estrogen produced by the ovaries may be reduced in premenopausal women who smoke. In 1982, the *New England Journal of Medicine* reported that levels of the three major estrogens—estradiol, estrone, and estriol—were reduced during the second half of the menstrual cycle in women who smoked. Another study in 1986 found evidence that women who smoke could not make estrogen in the ovaries with the same efficiency as nonsmokers.

Smoking's profound effect on the ovaries has been suggested by other studies that have examined the ages women who smoke become menopausal compared with women who do not smoke. The average age that American women become menopausal (between 50 and 52) has changed very little over the centuries. However, women who smoke become menopausal almost 2 years earlier than those who do not smoke. Perhaps even more distressing is the finding that women who do not smoke but who must regularly breathe the smoke of others also experience menopause about 2 years earlier! The reasons for early ovarian failure are not entirely clear, but it has been suggested that smoking destroys the eggs within the ovaries, leading to an earlier menopause.

In the premenopausal woman then, smoking may (1) decrease the production of estrogen in the ovaries, (2) cause estrogen to be changed chemically in the liver rendering it useless, and (3) cause an earlier menopause and total cessation of estrogen production in the ovaries.

What is the result of all these altered biochemical processes? Premenopausal women who smoke are estrogen deficient when compared with their nonsmoking premenopausal counterparts. And women who smoke or who are chronically exposed to the cigarette smoke of others become absolutely estrogen deficient 2 years earlier than average. The effect on the bone is premature and unnecessary bone loss. Ultimately, women who smoke or who are exposed to secondhand cigarette smoke find themselves at increased risk of osteoporotic fractures.

SMOKING AND POSTMENOPAUSAL ESTROGEN REPLACEMENT

Postmenopausal women have very low levels of estrogens in their blood since estrogen is no longer being produced by the ovaries. In studies that have measured estrogen levels in postmenopausal women who smoke and those who do not, no difference in the very low levels in both groups has been found. But there may be a very important effect of smoking in postmenopausal women who take oral estrogen replacement.

In 1992, researchers reported in the *Annals of Internal Medicine* that while estrogen replacement appeared to protect postmenopausal women from hip fractures, postmenopausal women who smoked were not protected if they took oral estrogen replacement. Estrogen pills are absorbed from the intestinal tract and almost immediately enter the circulation that passes through the liver. In women who smoke, the estrogen from the pill changes in the liver into the undesirable form of estrogen just as is the naturally produced estrogen in premenopausal women who smoke. This estrogen is not available to protect the bones. This isn't just a theory. Estrogen levels in smokers taking estrogen replacement have been found to be significantly lower than in nonsmokers taking estrogen replacement.

It would seem clear that smoking has the potential to harm the bones through its undesirable effects on the production and handling of estrogen by the body. The remedy would also seem equally clear. Don't smoke. If you already smoke, stop. And don't be shy about asking those around you who smoke to go elsewhere. It's your health that's on the line here.

COFFEE, TEA, COLA ANYONE?

I started drinking coffee when I was about 6 years old. My mother put a little coffee in my milk every morning. At some point in time, although I really don't remember when, I started putting a little milk in my coffee. I like coffee. I also can't seem to get started in the morning without it. I only need one cup, but heaven help anyone who comes between me and my morning cup of coffee.

I share that with you to reassure you that I am not going to suggest that you give up coffee, tea, colas, or any other caffeinated beverages. At least, I am not going to suggest that you give them up completely. A little moderation, however, is in order.

The potential culprit here is not the coffee or tea, but the caffeine they contain. Caffeine is a naturally occurring substance that is found in the leaves, seeds, or fruit of 63 different types of plants. Coffee beans, cocoa beans, tea leaves, and cola nuts are the most familiar sources of caffeine. In chemical terms, caffeine is an alkaloid. That means that it is an organic compound with alkaline properties. Caffeine comes from a chemical family known as methylxanthines. The point is, although caffeine occurs naturally in many beverages, it is a chemical. You could also consider it a drug. So it's not surprising that it has chemical or druglike effects on the human body. For the heart and brain, caffeine is a stimulant. That's why many people, myself included, find that a cup of coffee helps them wake up in the morning. There is actually a disease called caffeinism, which, as you might guess, refers to nervousness and sleeplessness brought on by consuming too much caffeine.

Caffeine's connection with osteoporosis is through calcium. We lose anywhere from 100 to 250 mg of calcium through the kidneys into the urine each day. Because most women become calcium deficient as teenagers, anything that increases the loss of calcium into the urine is going to magnify the calcium deficiency that most of us already have. Even if you are fortunate enough to have a diet that supplies adequate calcium, anything that increases your calcium losses into the urine will tip the scales toward calcium deficiency.

Caffeine has come under scrutiny because research has suggested that it can actually increase the amount of calcium lost into the urine each day. When you realize that many of us stop drinking beverage milk, our most concentrated calcium source, and replace milk with coffee, tea, or caffeinated colas, you realize that this could be a "double whammy" for our bones.

In 1982, Dr. Robert Heaney from Creighton University in Nebraska reported the results of a study of 170 postmenopausal women who consumed more than 1,000 mg of caffeine a day. One thousand mg of caffeine is the equivalent of about ten cups of coffee. Dr. Heaney found that this amount of caffeine could have a markedly undesirable effect on a woman's calcium metabolism. In another study of women ages 22 to 30, only 300 mg of caffeine caused the amount of calcium normally lost in the urine to double for the first 3 hours after drinking the caffeinated coffee. These same effects were confirmed in men as well. Three hundred mg of caffeine is equivalent to only three regular-sized cups of coffee. These research studies clearly raised the concern that caffeine could increase our calcium deficiency and contribute to the development of osteoporosis.

As these early research studies were evaluated, researchers raised two important additional questions: Did the loss of calcium caused by caffeine last all day or for only the first 3 hours after caffeine was ingested, and did it make any difference if one consumed a high-calcium diet or a low-calcium diet? Dr. Linda Massey, who had performed some of the early research on caffeine and calcium, concluded that caffeine did not cause significant calcium loss if the individual consumed at least 600 mg of calcium a day.

One of the best and most recent studies on caffeine's effects on calcium loss in women was published in 1990, again by Dr. Heaney and his colleagues Dr. Barger-Lux and Dr. Stegman. In this study, 16 healthy women were given 4 caffeine tablets per day. Each tablet contained 100 mg of caffeine for a total of 400 mg per day. They took these tablets every day for 19 days. None of the women in the study had calcium intakes less than 600 mg a day. They also took a multivitamin to provide vitamin D. The physicians measured the amount of calcium lost into the urine for 12 days while the women took the caffeine.

At the end of the study, Dr. Heaney and his colleagues could not show any harmful effect of this amount of caffeine on the amount of calcium lost into the urine. They concluded that 400 mg of caffeine did not appear to be harmful if the calcium intake was at least 600 mg a day. They also speculated that the increased loss of calcium in the urine after drinking caffeinated coffee may have only occurred for the first 3 hours and did not persist for the rest of the day.

A good, reasonable rule of thumb is to limit your consumption of caffeinated beverages, regardless of what they are, to no more than two servings per day. Then, drink decaffeinated.

Applying this research to our daily lives to help us reduce the risk of osteoporosis is fairly straightforward. The important message here is to get your calcium intake up and limit your caffeine intake to 400 mg or less a day.

So how much caffeine is in that cup of coffee anyway? Or in the cup of tea or can of cola? Some general statements are in order here before we get down to specifics. First, coffee will generally contain the most caffeine when compared with tea, colas, or cocoa. A cup of coffee will generally have two to three times as much caffeine as a cup of tea. The exact amount of caffeine in coffee or tea is quite variable. It depends upon the kind of bean or leaf used, the area where the plant was grown, the grind of the coffee, and the brewing time. With that in mind, I can only give you reasonable ranges for different types of coffee and tea. Cola and Dr. Pepper soft drinks obtain some of their caffeine content from the cola nut. The majority of the caffeine in these soft drinks is actually added and is obtained from the caffeine of decaffeinated raw coffee beans. Because of strict quality controls on the manufacture of soft drinks, the amount of caffeine in these beverages is consistently known. If you drink a mug of coffee instead of a cup, you must increase the caffeine content accordingly. A cup is about 5 ounces. Most mugs will hold about 10 ounces.

I can well imagine that right about now you are thinking that this is just one more thing to count. After all, most of us are counting calories. We have all been advised to count the milligrams of cholesterol and the grams of fat in our diets. I have certainly stressed to you the need to count your milligrams of calcium. Do you really need to count the milligrams of caffeine in your diet, too? No, I don't think so. Life shouldn't have to be so hard. A good, reasonable rule of thumb here is to limit your consumption of caffeinated beverages, regardless of what they are, to no more than two servings per day. Then, drink decaffeinated. As long as you are getting adequate calcium in your diet, this amount of caffeine should be safe.

CAFFEINE CONTENT IN COMMON BEVERAGES	
Coffee (5 ounces)	
Drip	110–150 mg
Percolated	64–124 mg
Instant	40–108 mg
Decaffeinated	2–5 mg
Instant decaffeinated	2 mg
Tea (5 ounces, bags or leaves)	
1-minute brew time	9–33 mg
3-minute brew time	20–46 mg
5-minute brew time	20–50 mg
Instant tea (5 ounces)	12–28 mg
Iced tea (12 ounces)	22–36 mg
Cocoa (5 ounces)	4 mg
Chocolate milk (8 ounces)	5 mg
Soft drinks (12 ounces)	
Coca Cola	45.6 mg
Dr. Pepper	39.6 mg
Pepsi-Cola	38.4 mg
Big Red	38.4 mg
RC Cola	36.0 mg
Shasta Cola	44.4 mg
Mr. Pibb	40.8 mg
Mountain Dew	54.0 mg
Root beer	0 mg

Source: U.S. Food and Drug Administration and National Soft Drink Association.

CHAPTER 6

Exercise and Osteoporosis

The idea that exercise plays a role in the development of strong bones is not new. In fact, it's ridiculously old. In 1892, a German named Wolff theorized that the bones became stronger in response to increased exercise, which would make the bones less likely to fracture. Wolff's theory, as it has come to be called, is accepted as fact today. But how do we know?

Early knowledge about the effects of exercise on the development and maintenance of the bones came from observations of individuals at opposite extremes: individuals who were totally inactive and individuals who were world-class athletes.

In the early 1970s researchers reported on the effects of bedrest on calcium and bone. In one study, 3 men remained at complete bedrest for 30 to 36 weeks. Calcium was lost from the bodies of these men at a rate of 0.5% to 0.7% every month. After 36 weeks of bedrest, 25% to 45% of the bone was lost from the heel. In a second study, 5 men maintained bedrest for 20 to 30 weeks with a similar loss of calcium from the body. In 1983, another group of scientists measured the spinal bone density in patients put to bed for an average of 27 days because of herniated discs. These patients lost an average of 0.9% of their bone from the spine every week while they remained at bedrest. In a sense, these results were not surprising. Physicians had observed that patients who were paralyzed or who remained in bed for long periods of time due to illness had

less bone on X rays. What was surprising in these research studies was how fast this happens even in otherwise healthy people. With these types of studies, the scientists were also able to prove that it was the inactivity itself that caused the bone loss and not a disease.

For additional proof, a more extreme example of nonuse of the bones occurs during space flight. In the absence of gravity, the bones have very little to do. They no longer must support the weight of the body even at rest. The astronauts in the Gemini space program lost significant amounts of bone during their space flights as did the astronauts from the space station Skylab. This confirmed Wolff's theory that the amount and strength of the bone are directly linked to the amount of activity that forces the bones to bear weight and move against resistance.

If activity and exercise are such important factors, we would expect world-class athletes to have bigger and stronger bones. A report from Sweden in 1971 examined the bone density in the thighs of 64 world-class athletes. Among these athletes, there were 11 weight lifters, 25 runners, 15 soccer players, 9 swimmers, and 4 throwers. These men were compared with 24 healthy men who exercised for fitness and 15 men who did not exercise at all. As you might expect, all the athletes had a higher bone density than the nonathletes. The nonathletes who exercised had a higher bone density than the nonexercising

nother study of
, the racket arm
greater bone
ket arm. This
he theory that
                 n, not made.

fc   re required
to   ... the development of a
greater bone density. Incredible forces are
certainly generated during the type of
weight lifting that professional weight
lifters do.

In another study, also from Sweden, physicians found that the bone density in the lumbar spine in professional weight lifters was directly related to the amount of weight they lifted during training. These were men capable of lifting over 600 lbs.! While the ability to lift 600 lbs. is not too relevant to you or me, these athletes illustrate the other extreme of activity and weight bearing for the skeleton.

Critics of studies in world-class athletes argued that the sport did not make the bones strong. Indeed, they said that these athletes inherited the strong bones. That might be partially true. Perhaps the most telling evidence that proves that the sport makes the bones strong has come from studying tennis players. Tennis is a good sport for this type of study because both legs are used equally in the sport, but only one arm is really involved. The arm that holds the racket is the only one that receives the impact of the ball and the force of the swing. There are no medical findings to suggest that one arm could inherit a better ability to make bone than the other arm. So scientists measured the bone strength in different groups of tennis players. In one study of college women, the racket arm was found to have 16% greater bone mineral than

The studies in athletes from different sports also clearly suggest that some sports have more bone-building potential than others. In the study I discussed above, the weight lifters had the best bone strength in the leg, followed by the runners and soccer players. The swimmers, although they did have better bone in the legs than the nonexercising group, were not better by much. Other studies in swimmers have found the bones in the spine to be no better than in people who don't exercise at all. Why? After all, swimming is great for your heart and lungs. So why isn't it a good bone exercise?

The water, not your bones, supports the body's weight while you are swimming. Swimming, then, is not a weight-bearing activity. Swimming is also not an impact-loading sport for the bones. Impact loading means that a force is being transmitted to the bones from an external source. The impact of the foot striking the ground during running, for example, is impact loading. In weight lifting, the bones of the legs and spine must support the weight of the object being lifted. They are loaded with this extra weight in addition to supporting the weight of the body against gravity. There is no impact loading and no weight bearing in swimming. As a consequence, swimmers may be very fit from the standpoint of cardiovascular endurance, but they do not obtain significant bone benefits from their sport.

Another observation from studies in athletes is that the bones benefit from exercise only if they are used in the exercise. That makes perfect sense of course.

But early in our research, it was actually common for researchers to have people exercise by running and then see what effect the running might have had on the arm bone density. That may sound strange but the thinking was that exercise might cause the body to produce some type of hormone or other substance that would have a general effect on all of the bones in the body, not just the ones that were being exercised.

Not surprisingly, studies of the arm bones in runners did not show that running had any beneficial effect on the arm. The studies on the arms of tennis players demonstrated that the nonracket arm had only an average bone density, while the racket arm had an increased bone density. The arm that was not being used in the activity did not benefit. Exercise is site specific. If you want a strong spine, you must exercise the spine. If you want strong legs, you must exercise the legs.

Exercise is site specific. If you want a strong spine you must exercise the spine. If you want strong legs, you must exercise the legs.

Another rather obvious difference between weight lifters and runners is in the amount of muscle that the two groups have. Weight lifters must of necessity have large, well-developed muscles. Runners, on the other hand, are usually slender individuals and are not generally characterized as having large amounts of muscle. Could the difference in muscle size and strength have any relationship to the strength or density of the bones?

There are several research studies that suggest that muscle strength does have a direct bearing on bone strength. It appears that not only does the bone respond to the amount of weight it must support, it also responds to the force of the muscle pulling on it. The stronger the muscle, the more forceful the pull on the bone to which it is attached and—viola!—the stronger the bone. Let me reassure you now, however, that you don't have to become a power lifter with huge muscles to strengthen your bones.

A reasonable question at this point is to ask, "Is it ever too late to start an exercise program to prevent osteoporosis?" The answer is definitely no, but the sooner you start, the better.

EFFECT OF EXERCISE ON PEAK BONE MASS

Left to its own devices, the body does the vast majority of its bone building in the first 30 years of life. In fact, most of the bone strength in the spine is probably acquired by the time we're 20. We may have a little longer to develop the strength in the bone in our legs. Research that looks at the effects of exercise on the bone in growing youngsters is relatively new. The older techniques used to measure bone density involved too much radiation exposure to use in healthy children. With the newer techniques available now, these studies are being done. To no one's surprise, researchers are finding that boys and girls who are more physically active develop stronger bones.

A revealing study from the University of Indiana in 1991 looked at the relationship between the hours children spent participating in different sports and the amount of bone in their arms and legs. There was a strong relationship between the total hours spent being active and the bone strength in the forearm and hip regions. The type of activity also seemed to

make a difference. Children who participated in weight-bearing activities like
baseball, soccer, basketball, and tennis
demonstrated a positive relationship
between the time spent in those activities
and the amount of bone they had. In other
words, the more time spent, the greater
their bone strength. On the other hand,
children who participated in nonweight-
bearing sports, like biking and swimming,
had a negative relationship. The more time
spent in those activities, the lower the bone
strength. The conclusion that one would
draw from this is that our children need to
be doing weight-bearing exercise to help
them achieve their maximum potential to
build bone. Every increase in the peak
bone mass developed by our children will
result in fewer osteoporotic fractures as
adults. There is, however, one caveat. The
enhancement of peak bone mass will only
be of real benefit if this bone mass is maintained into adult life. Can exercise maintain bone after the ripe old age of 20?

EFFECT OF EXERCISE IN PREMENOPAUSAL WOMEN

We tend to think of bone as simply the
structural support for the body. This creates the impression that bone, like the steel
supports of a large building, is just a hard
substance with no life of its own. Bone is
alive. Bone responds to its environment by
changing in strength or density and even
shape. We can still influence the strength
of the bone with exercise as mature adults.
If we become inactive as mature adults, we
will lose bone strength. If we stay active,
we can maintain the bone strength we
achieved as youngsters. Even if we weren't
active as youngsters, the bones will respond to exercise with a maintenance or
an increase in strength if we begin an exercise program as adults.

EFFECT OF EXERCISE IN POSTMENOPAUSAL WOMEN

More research on the benefits of exercise
for the bones has been done in postmenopausal women than in premenopausal
women. Many of these studies asked postmenopausal women, who did not exercise
regularly, to participate in different types
of exercise programs for 1 to 2 years. The
bone density was measured at the beginning of the study and again at the end.
Researchers were also interested in
whether these women were taking estrogen replacement during the study.

In 1988 in the *Annals of Internal
Medicine,* Dr. Gail Dalsky, an exercise
physiologist, reported that postmenopausal women who did 50 to 60 minutes
of weight-bearing exercise 3 times a week
increased their spinal bone content by
5.2% after only 9 months. These women
had been inactive prior to beginning the
program and only a few were taking estrogen. Their average age was 62. At the end
of 22 months, the bone content increased
6.1%. A similar group of women who did
not exercise but were simply observed during the study, lost 1.1% during the same
period of time. The types of exercises used
in this study were brisk walking, jogging,
and stair climbing—all weight-bearing,
impact-loading exercises.

In 1992, in the *Journal of Bone
and Mineral Research,* Dr. Leslie Pruitt
reported on a study involving postmenopausal women not taking estrogen
replacement who participated in a weight-
training program for 9 months. These
women exercised 3 times a week for 1 hour
using dumbbells, ankle weights, and Universal gym equipment. Their average age
was 54. After 9 months, the average gain
in the spine bone density was 1.6% while
a similar group of women in the study
who did not exercise lost 3.6%. The

exercising group also had a small gain in the wrist bone strength while the sedentary group had a small loss. Dr. Pruitt was not able to show any difference in the two groups in the hip region of the leg. The importance of this study is that although the gain in the spine bone density was small, these women did gain! They did not lose bone in the spine like their nonexercising counterparts even though none of them was taking estrogen to help protect their bones.

To take things one step further, a study from Florida looked at the effect of weight training on postmenopausal women who were taking estrogen. These women were in their mid- to late forties. They exercised for about 20 minutes, 3 days a week for 1 year using Nautilus equipment. The bone density or strength in their spines and forearms was measured at the beginning and at the end of the exercise study. The results were compared with another group of women who were also taking estrogen but who did not exercise. The women taking estrogen but not exercising did not lose bone during the year-long study. The women who were taking estrogen *and* exercising gained 8.3% in their spines and 4.1% in the forearms. This study suggests that not only is exercise beneficial, the addition of estrogen replacement to exercise or exercise to estrogen replacement (depending upon your point of view) is even better.

Even in studies where the researchers could not demonstrate dramatic gains in bone with exercise, researchers have been able to show that exercise slows bone loss. At the University of Wisconsin, Dr. Everett Smith and his colleagues studied women for 4 years. The average age of these women was 50. Slightly less than half of these women were postmenopausal when they began the program. Exercising for 45 minutes, 3 days a week, these women performed activities that included dancing, walking, and jogging during the first year. As the study progressed, the women also used light weights and elastic tubing to provide resistance for some exercises. The forearm and upper arm were measured in this study. A similar group of women who were not exercising was followed for the sake of comparison. Although gains in bone were not demonstrated in this study, the exercising group lost significantly less bone than the nonexercisers. This was true whether the women were pre- or postmenopausal. The intensity of this exercise program was rather mild when compared with the other studies, but it was effective in retarding bone loss.

EFFECT OF EXERCISE IN WOMEN WITH OSTEOPOROSIS

Women who have lost enough bone to be said to have osteoporosis but who have not had fractures are not really included in this category in exercise research studies. In this instance, this refers to women who have already broken bones because of osteoporosis. There are many benefits of exercise in this group that go beyond the bones. Relief of pain; improvement in posture, muscle strength, tone, agility, and balance; and a reduction in the risk of falling can all come from exercise. And, yes, bone loss can be slowed as well and, no, it doesn't matter how old you are.

One of the tragic consequences of having an osteoporotic fracture is that so often the pain forces a woman to spend weeks or months in bed. The longer she remains inactive, the more weakened the muscles become, making activity more difficult. At bedrest, the bones actually begin to lose even more calcium, which makes the disease worse. As the back muscles weaken, the spine tends to curve forward because the strength is not there to hold the spine erect. This actually forces the spine into a posture that makes it more susceptible to fractures in the future. (This also contributes to the dowager's hump that women with osteoporosis develop.) With inactivity comes generalized muscle weakness, poor endurance, and decreased agility, all of which combine to increase the risk of falling. Some women have even been advised not to exercise after an osteoporotic fracture for fear that exercise will cause more fractures. The concern is valid. Some types of exercise would increase a woman's risk for additional fractures but no exercise only perpetuates the osteoporosis and will result in an overall decline in health. The key is to exercise safely.

> *Some women have been advised not to exercise after an osteoporotic fracture . . . but no exercise only perpetuates the osteoporosis and will result in an overall decline in health.*

The woman with osteoporosis can exercise safely, but there are activities and exercises she must avoid. Any activity that requires repeated forward bending from the waist with the back rounded (called trunk flexion) may increase the risk of spinal fracture. This would include toe-touches or sit-ups. High-impact activities, like running or rope jumping, could place too much stress on the weakened spine, causing it to collapse. She must also avoid activities, like skiing, skating, or exercising on slippery floors, that increase her likelihood of falling. Safe and beneficial exercises include back-extension exercises in which the back is arched. Low-impact, weight-bearing activity, such as walking, is also both desirable and safe. Even weights or exercise machines can be safely utilized—regardless of age—with great benefit to the woman with osteoporosis.

TYPES OF WEIGHT-BEARING ACTIVITY

Weight-bearing activity in general can be thought of as any activity that you do on your feet, requiring your bones to support the weight of your body against gravity. Impact-loading, weight-bearing activity would involve some impact or force being transmitted to the skeleton during weight bearing. Weight bearing and impact loading stimulate the development of good healthy bones. Some types of weight-bearing, impact-loading activities are characterized as aerobic and some are anaerobic. Let's look at what these terms mean and how they might affect your choice of activity.

AEROBIC EXERCISE

Aerobic exercise means that the energy needed for the muscles to work is produced from fat, protein, and carbohydrates that have been combined with oxygen. For almost any sort of sustained muscular activity lasting more than 3 minutes in length, the muscles utilize this oxygen-based fuel production for energy.

For an activity or exercise to be considered aerobic, it must be rhythmic, use large muscles, and be continuous in nature. The largest muscles in the body are found in the legs and back. These large muscles must be used continuously and rhythmically, not in a jerky, intermittent fashion for the activity to be aerobic.

Most activities that end in "ing" are aerobic exercises. Running, jogging, bicycling, swimming, and dancing are examples of sports that are aerobic. But remember, the aerobic exercise of swimming is not weight bearing or impact loading. There is no such thing as "basketballing" or "baseballing" or "tennising." These sports are not aerobic, although they are weight bearing and may be impact loading in nature. (They are not aerobic because the movements are not continuous.) There are, of course, exceptions to the "ing" rule. Bowling is not considered an aerobic exercise. And, in my experience, someone always asks if sky diving is aerobic. It's not, but it certainly can be impact loading!

Most activities that end in "ing" (such as bicycling) are aerobic.

ANAEROBIC EXERCISE

In anaerobic exercise, the muscles do not use oxygen to produce the fuel they need. Instead, the fuel is produced from substances called ATP and CP, which are stored in small amounts in the muscles. In anaerobic exercise, the fuel can also be produced from glucose. Brief but very strenuous exercise is anaerobic exercise. The body can quickly convert ATP to fuel for the sudden bursts of energy that are needed in a 100-yard dash or a quick run down the basketball court. Glucose can also be turned into fuel a little more quickly than carbohydrates or fat combined with oxygen. Some activities are strictly aerobic, others are anaerobic, and some are both.

If you are going to do weight-bearing, impact-loading exercise for your bones, you might as well perform an *aero-bic* weight-bearing, impact-loading activity in order to obtain the cardiovascular benefits from the exercise as well.

THE CARDIOVASCULAR BENEFITS OF AEROBIC EXERCISE

As living creatures that require oxygen to sustain life, we must be able to take the oxygen from the air we breathe and then deliver it to the various tissues in the body. This isn't as easy as it sounds. Getting oxygen from the air to the organs of the body is a complex process that involves the lungs, heart, and blood vessels working together. With each breath we take, the lungs must extract the oxygen from the air. The oxygen then passes across barriers in the lung into the bloodstream. Blood that is initially low in oxygen is pumped from the heart into the lungs to receive the oxygen. The blood carries the oxygen attached to hemoglobin, which is a component of the red blood cells. Once the blood receives its load of oxygen, it returns to the heart to be circulated to the rest of the body. For this phase to work with maximum efficiency, the heart muscle must contract forcefully and efficiently, ejecting the blood into the general circulation. Once the oxygenated blood arrives at the muscles or other tissue that need the oxygen, the oxygen is removed from the blood by the tissue. The blood then returns to the heart to be sent to the lungs again for more oxygen. Aerobic exercise improves the efficiency with which we can do all this.

In judging how aerobically fit an individual is or how demanding an aerobic activity may be, doctors often use two measures of aerobic work. One measure uses a concept called "METS." The other measure uses the concept of the "target heart rate."

METS stands for metabolic equivalents. It is a measure of how much oxygen is used by the body during an activity. An activity that requires one MET of work means that during that activity, your body needs 3.5 milliliters (ml) of oxygen every minute for every 2.2 lbs. that you weigh. Another way of looking at an individual's aerobic fitness or at the demands of an exercise is the VO_2 max. This is the maximum amount of oxygen an individual is capable of utilizing during an activity. Your VO_2 max is determined by how efficiently your lungs can extract oxygen from the air and pass it into the bloodstream and by how efficiently your heart can pump the oxygenated blood to the rest of the body. For example, if you performed an activity that required your body to use 35 ml of oxygen every minute for each 2.2 lbs. of body weight, your VO_2 max is 35 ml/min/2.2 lbs. The VO_2 max could also be said to be 10 METS (since 1 MET is 3.5 ml/min/2.2 lbs., 35 ml/min/2.2 lbs. would equal 10 METS). You have probably heard athletes say, "I had to stop because I ran out of air." What they are really saying is that they reached their VO_2 max and it wasn't good enough to provide sufficient oxygen for them to continue exercising at that intensity.

Although you now know how many METS on average an activity may require, a more convenient gauge of how hard you are actually working during an aerobic activity is your heart rate. This is why many people use a "target heart rate" to guide them in performing aerobic exercise. Your maximum heart rate and your VO_2 max are closely related. In a healthy individual, the heart rate goes up as the oxygen consumption or VO_2 max goes up. As we get older, the maximum heart rate we can sustain goes down. You can predict your maximum heart rate with following equation:

AVERAGE NUMBER OF METS REQUIRED BY DIFFERENT ACTIVITIES

Activity	Average METS
Golf (walking)	5.1
Handball	10
Judo	13.5
Jumping rope (70 skips/min)	9
Bicycling 10 mph	7
Running 6-minute mile	16.3
Walking 3 mph	3.3
Jogging 5 mph	8.6
Swimming	6
Stair climbing	6
Cross-country skiing	10
Shuffleboard	2.5
Fishing	3.7
Racquetball	9
Handball	10
Sitting in a chair	1
Sleeping	< 1
Skating	6.5
Soccer	8.5

Predicted Maximum Heart Rate $=$ 220 − Your Age

If you are 35 years old, your maximum heart rate is 220 − 35, or 185 beats per minute. When you are exercising aerobically to improve your cardiovascular fitness, you want to exercise with enough intensity to reach what is called the target heart rate range. The target heart rate range is 70% to 90% of your predicted maximum heart rate. For the 35-year-old with a predicted maximum heart rate of 185, the 70% to 90% range is 129 to 166 beats per minute. Exercising in this range is expected to dramatically improve the efficiency with which your heart can pump blood and the efficiency with which your lungs extract oxygen from the air. The result will be an improvement in your VO$_2$ max. As your heart and lungs function more efficiently, you will find that your resting heart rate actually slows down. You will breathe more efficiently and your heart will beat more efficiently. As a result, you can deliver the same amount of oxygen to your body as you did before with fewer heartbeats per minute.

As you become more fit, you will have to exercise with more intensity to get your heart rate into the target range. You will have to increase the METS of your activity. The specific number of METS any individual uses during an activity will vary depending on the effort she exerts and, for sports, the level of skill she possesses.

How quickly you improve your fitness level, or VO$_2$ max, will depend on your initial level of fitness and how often, how hard, and how long you exercise. In general, if you exercise very hard at the upper end of the target heart rate range, you can exercise for shorter periods of time and see gains in your fitness level. I generally don't recommend this approach, however, because it increases your risk of injury. Exercising at low to moderate intensities, or toward the lower end of your target heart rate range for longer periods of time, will also improve your fitness level equally well with less risk of injury. It may not seem fair, but people who are the least fit will make larger gains more quickly than people who are already reasonably fit when they start a program. However, good gains can be expected by everyone in the first 6 to 8 weeks of a program. Once you have reached a desired level of fitness, you have to keep exercising to keep that level.

An exercise intensity that brings your heart rate to 70% of your maximum predicted heart rate is required to maintain fitness. You will need to exercise at this level 3 times a week in order to avoid what is called "deconditioning," or the loss of fitness and a decline in your new VO$_2$ max.

For the healthy woman who has no restrictions on her ability to exercise, the concept of METS and a target heart rate range is used as a guide to determine how hard she must exercise to obtain the cardiovascular benefits of aerobic exercise. For an older individual who may have health problems that limit the intensity with which she can exercise safely, METS and a target heart rate range are often used as limits that the individual should not exceed for safety reasons.

TYPES OF STRENGTH TRAINING

Strength training or resistance training can be divided into three basic types: isotonic, isokinetic, and isometric. Most of the exercise performed in strength training is isotonic exercise. Isokinetic exercise is performed infrequently. The prefix "iso" means equal. So isotonic means "same tone," isokinetic means "same speed," and isometric means "same length." These terms describe what happens to the muscles during the exercise. Free weights or dumbbells, ankle and wrist weights, weight machines, and even elastic tubing can be used for strength training.

ISOTONIC STRENGTH-TRAINING EXERCISES

A strength-training exercise that was described as isotonic meant that during the exercise the tone of the muscle or the tension being generated by the muscles remained the same throughout the entire range of motion through which the weight was lifted. We know now that the tension in the muscle does change as a weight is lifted. As a consequence, the term isotonic exercise has taken on a slightly new meaning and implies that the weight or resistance against which the muscle is working remains constant. The length of the muscle changes during the exercise, shortening as the weight is lifted and lengthening as the weight is lowered. The speed during lifting and lowering of the weight may also vary. Exercises using free weights (dumbbells) and resistance machines (Nautilus, Universal, or Cybex) are isotonic strength-training exercises. Some exercise experts prefer to call this type of exercise "dynamic constant resistance exercise" rather than isotonic since the tone in the muscle does not remain the same but the resistance or weight does.

ISOKINETIC STRENGTH-TRAINING EXERCISE

Isokinetic strength-training exercise describes resistance exercise in which the muscle moves at a constant speed. The force the muscle is working against can vary. Clearly the length of the muscle varies as it contracts and relaxes. Isokinetic exercise has gained in popularity over the last few years for several reasons. Theoretically, it is a safer form of exercise than isotonic exercise using dumbbells or isotonic machines.

The reason this type of exercise is considered safer is that the machine only gives you as much resistance as you give it. For example, on isokinetic machines designed to exercise the long back extensor muscles, the muscles that go up and down

on either side of the spine, an individual pushes backwards on a padded bar that lays across the back at shoulder-blade level. The harder she pushes, the harder the machines pushes back. So the machine will never give her more resistance than she can handle. Injuries due to muscle strain from attempting to lift a weight that's too heavy on an isotonic machine are much less likely to occur on an isokinetic machine.

The other advantage to isokinetics is that the speed of the exercise is controlled. This makes it possible to exercise at faster speeds than are generally possible with an isotonic machine with less chance of injury. Isokinetic machines are not commonly available in most clubs. The large machines tend to be very expensive. Some manufacturers have recently introduced reasonably priced home isokinetic machines. Fortunately for our purposes, isotonic training and isometric training will suffice nicely.

ISOMETRIC STRENGTH-TRAINING EXERCISE

The best way to understand isometric exercise is by imagining you are trying to push down a brick wall with one arm. The wall doesn't move (obviously) even though you are pushing with all your might. The muscles in your arm are attempting to contract with tremendous force, but they can't because the wall is simply too heavy to move. So the muscle stays the same length. That's isometric exercise. You can gain muscle strength with isometric exercise and it has the added benefit of requiring little if any equipment (all you need, for example, is a brick wall). I use isometric exercise primarily to strengthen the stomach muscles in an individual who has any type of back problem, including those caused by osteoporosis. I otherwise prefer isotonic strength training to isometrics. The reason is simply that I want the muscle to lengthen and shorten completely, because this puts a more varied and dynamic strain on the bones. I need that dynamic strain to increase bone strength. In older individuals, or anyone with high blood pressure, I also would rather not use isometrics because there is a greater tendency to elevate the blood pressure with this type of strength training.

BEFORE YOU BEGIN
ANY EXERCISE PROGRAM . . .

Anyone who recommends any kind of exercise program always says something like "Consult your physician before beginning an exercise program" or "If you are over 40, see your doctor before beginning an exercise program." When I was in my twenties and thirties, I always felt comfortable ignoring such advice because I knew I was basically healthy and my forties seemed like a very long way away. Now that I am past forty, my initial reaction to such advice is to find it insulting. After all, what magically happens at 40 that wasn't true at 39? Forty is hardly over the hill! But the reality is that after the age of 40, your body can change in ways that might affect your ability to safely perform part or all of an exercise program. There are things that might specifically affect your ability to exercise safely that only your doctor knows. Above all, I want you to exercise safely. So when do you need to see a doctor before beginning an exercise program?

The American College of Sports Medicine developed recommendations for medical evaluations and testing that should be done before an individual begins

an exercise program. The College states that *"women who are 50 years of age, or younger, who are apparently healthy,"* do not absolutely need a medical examination or testing prior to beginning an exercise program. Healthy women over 50 who are beginning a moderately strenuous exercise program also do not absolutely need an evaluation before starting. If the exercise program is a vigorous one, then healthy women over 50 should see their physicians first.

So how does a moderate exercise program differ from a vigorous one? A moderate program is one that begins and proceeds gradually, remaining well within the individual's current capacity to perform. This means you should be able to comfortably sustain the exercise for 60 minutes. This type of exercise requires that you exert yourself at about 40% to 60% of your maximum capabilities. An individual who is *just beginning* an exercise program generally cannot exercise vigorously for more than 15 or 20 minutes. Maintaining vigorous exercise requires that you work at more than 60% of your current capacity. So how do you know what your capacity is? We use the METS and target heart rates concepts to figure it out. You really can't know what your actual capacity is without some very fancy medical testing, because doctors are using the VO_2 max as a base for these guidelines. So instead, we use a maximum heart rate, based on age, as a guide. Use the formula for predicting your maximum heart rate (220 − Your Age). A moderate exercise program would increase your heart rate 40% to 60% of your maximum predicted heart rate, while a vigorous exercise program would increase your heart rate above 60% of your predicted maximum heart rate. So if you are 55, your predicted maximum heart rate is 220 − 55, or 165 beats per minute. Sixty percent of your maximum heart rate is 99 beats per minute. If your exercise program begins and progresses gradually and your heart rate does not initially exceed 99 beats per minute, the exercise program would be classified as moderate. If your heart rate goes over 99 beats per minute while you are exercising, you must consider the program vigorous.

The American College of Sports Medicine also points out that individuals of *any* age who have two or more risk factors for heart disease or symptoms of heart, lung, liver, kidney, or thyroid disease or who have diabetes should absolutely be evaluated by a physician before beginning a vigorous exercise program. Those individuals with only risks and no symptoms do not necessarily have to see a physician before beginning a moderate exercise program. The risk factors noted by the College include:

1. High blood pressure, even when treated with medication
2. Serum cholesterol level greater than 240 mg/dl
3. Cigarette smoking
4. Family history of heart disease in parents or siblings which occurred under the age of 55
5. Diabetes that does not require insulin for treatment

If two or more of these statements apply to you, you should see your doctor before beginning a vigorous exercise program regardless of your age.

Symptoms or signs of possible heart, lung, or organ disease, according to the American College of Sports Medicine include:

1. Chest pain, left arm pain, or neck pain that occurs with activity
2. Sudden shortness of breath or shortness of breath with activity

3. Dizziness or fainting
4. Shortness of breath while lying down
5. Swelling of the ankles
6. Palpitations
7. Pain in the legs while walking
8. Heart murmur

If you have *any* of these signs or symptoms, regardless of your age, you should see your doctor before beginning either a moderate or vigorous exercise program.

As you can see, the American College of Sports Medicine has concentrated on the individual who might have some type of heart, lung, or circulation problem. I am also concerned about the health of your bones and their safety during your exercise program. Could you have already experienced some bone loss that might make certain exercises hazardous for you? For any woman who is menopausal, this is an important question that should be answered before beginning an exercise program.

There are certain exercises that, while ordinarily beneficial, would potentially increase your risk of having a fracture if you have already lost a significant amount of bone. As a consequence, if you are menopausal and have not taken estrogen replacement for a year or more at any time since menopause, I recommend that you see your doctor, regardless of your age or the type of exercise program. Your physician may need a bone-density test to determine if you have lost enough bone to be at risk for fracture.

If you know that you have heart disease, lung disease, or any type of chronic medical problem, including osteoporosis, you should see your doctor before beginning an exercise program, regardless of your age. This does not mean that you cannot or should not exercise. It simply means that changes may need to be made to your exercise program to ensure your safety. After all, a doctor's most important rule in caring for patients is "First, do no harm." Your most important rule in beginning an exercise program should be, "First, don't injure myself."

MEDICATIONS AND EXERCISE

Almost all of us, at one time or another, have had to take medication to treat an illness or to relieve some type of unpleasant symptom. Some medications may affect your ability to exercise safely by altering the blood pressure or heart beat response to exercise. Absolutely do not stop any medication without the advice of your doctor. Review the lists of medications in the appendices. If you are taking any of these medications, talk to your doctor about your exercise program and how your medications might affect your response to exercise.

CAN YOU EXERCISE TOO MUCH?

Yes, you can. Women who exercise so strenuously that their menstrual periods become irregular or stop increase their risk of bone loss and osteoporosis. The function of the ovaries is impaired under these circumstances; estrogen levels fall, causing bone loss. Many women athletes do not realize that the welcome convenience of not having menstrual periods is actually a sign of potential disaster for the bones. Surprisingly, fractures can occur in these young women who are otherwise extreme-

ly fit. In competitive athletes, exercise-induced menstrual abnormalities can be difficult to treat. The most direct approach is to ask the athlete to reduce the intensity of her exercise and gain a small amount of weight. That is an unacceptable approach for most of these highly competitive women. As an alternative, physicians are prescribing the estrogens found in oral contraceptives in order to protect the bones of these young women. For the average woman who is not engaged in athletic competition, it is unlikely that exercise will be sufficiently strenuous to cause menstrual irregularities. If menstrual periods do become irregular or stop, you should reduce the intensity of your exercise program and see your doctor.

GET READY, GET SET . . .

I think it's about time we got started with an actual exercise program. Remember, in this program, my emphasis is on the prevention of osteoporosis. For that I need weight-bearing and strength-training exercises. I want to take advantage of the heart and lung benefits of aerobic exercise, too, so I will emphasize weight-bearing exercises that are aerobic in nature. Most of the strength training I recommend will be isotonic, but for individuals with osteoporosis or any type of back problem, we will use isometric exercises for the stomach muscles. In the next two chapters, I will outline some guiding exercise principles as well as specific programs for (1) the healthy woman exercising to prevent osteoporosis and (2) the woman with osteoporosis.

CHAPTER 7

Exercising to Prevent Osteoporosis

If you'll pardon the pun, the heart and soul of an exercise program to prevent osteoporosis are weight-bearing and strength-training exercises. Remember, weight-bearing exercise requires you to be on your feet so that your bones support the weight of your body against gravity. Activities such as walking, jogging, tennis, basketball, volleyball, baseball, and skating are all examples of weight-bearing exercise. Swimming is a nonweight-bearing exercise because the water—not the bones—supports the body's weight. Bicycling is somewhere in between. When you sit on the bicycle seat, your spine supports the weight of your upper body. But your legs rest on the pedals; they are not supporting your body weight. As a consequence, bicycling is weight bearing for the spine but not for your legs.

The addition of impact loading to weight-bearing exercise improves the bone benefits of the exercise. Just as it sounds, impact loading means that an impact or force is transmitted to the bones in the course of the activity. For example, when you walk at a casual pace, the impact or force of your heel striking the ground is equivalent to about 1.3 times the weight of your body. Walking at 3 mph increases the force on your heel to 1.5 times the weight of your body. When you pick up your pace to a jog of 7.5 to 10 mph, the force on your heel also increases to 5 times the weight of your body. Other activities like volleyball or skipping rope involve a significant amount of impact loading.

Exercises that combine weight bearing and impact loading can also be either aerobic or anaerobic. Jogging and running are clearly aerobic forms of exercise. Volleyball, although it is weight bearing and involves impact loading every time the player jumps up to spike a ball, is primarily an anaerobic exercise. Although both are beneficial for the bones, the greatest cardiovascular benefit will come from the aerobic exercise. If you like to play volleyball, tennis, racquetball, or any of a number of anaerobic weight-bearing sports, continue to do so by all means. These are excellent bone activities. However, exercise for the sake of exercise should be as efficient as we can make it. Aerobic, weight-bearing, impact-loading exercise combines the health benefits for the heart and the bones most efficiently.

STRENGTH TRAINING

An exercise program that relies solely on aerobic weight-bearing exercise is incomplete. The addition of strength training, preferably isotonic strength training, is an essential component in a complete osteoporosis-prevention exercise program. The phrase strength training implies that the purpose of this type of exercise is to increase muscle strength, but strength training strengthens the bones as well.

Women have tended to shy away from strength training in the past for fear of appearing unfeminine. Concern over the development of large muscles also persuaded many women to avoid this type of exercise. These fears are both unfounded and unfortunate. Strength training for women has the potential to have enormous health benefits. Strength training is the most efficient way to exercise a specific bone. Although running exercises the leg bones and the spine in terms of weight bearing and impact loading, the arm bones do not receive any benefit from this type of activity. When you run, the force on the lower spine is greater than on the middle or upper spine. Each area of the spine can be directly exercised with strength training. The recognition that strength training for women was an important aspect of exercise programs to prevent osteoporosis prompted the American College of Sports Medicine to add strength training to its exercise recommendations for women. The recommendations had previously only included aerobic weight-bearing activities.

Women also benefit from strength training in other ways. Improvement in muscle strength and tone is beneficial in a variety of ways. The most obvious benefit is a cosmetic one. You will have a nicer-looking figure if the muscles are firm. The line of the shoulders, arms, and legs is really much more attractive when the shape is determined by a firm muscle rather than a flabby muscle.

You will not develop big, bulging muscles from strength training. This has been such a concern that there have actually been research studies in which the dimensions of women's muscles have been measured before and after strength training programs to see how much change in size has occurred. In one study, which lasted 10 weeks, the largest change the researchers could measure in any muscle was an increase of 0.6 centimeters. That's about 1/4 of an inch. In this same study, the

dimensions of the hip, thighs, and stomach actually decreased 1/8 to 1/4 of an inch. Does anyone really object to that? Even the most intense strength-training programs do not produce marked increases in muscle size in women. In one 6-month program, a group of women athletes increased their upper body strength by 37%. The diameter of their upper arms increased by only 1/2 inch.

Our muscles do increase in strength in response to strength-training exercise, but they don't increase greatly in size for two apparent reasons. First, we don't have the hormones for it. The male sex hormone testosterone is largely responsible for the greater size of a man's muscles compared with that of a woman's. Although women do have small amounts of testosterone normally, it is not enough to produce large, bulky muscles. In addition, when women engage in strength training, a decrease in fat accompanies the increase in muscle. The end result is very little increase, if any, in overall size.

The other obvious benefit of strength-training exercise, particularly in the upper body, is the increase in muscle strength itself. Many women have very weak arms, shoulders, and upper backs. On average, we have only half of a man's strength in our arms while we have 75% of a man's strength in our legs. In one study, 40% of women in their fifties could not even lift 10 lbs. Sixty percent of women in their sixties and older could not lift 10 lbs. A reasonably strong upper body is necessary for many things that we do during the course of day in taking care of our homes, families, and jobs.

Another misconception about strength training is it reduces your flexibility. This is not true. When performed correctly, strength training can actually result in increased flexibility. Finally, even though strength training is considered an anaerobic form of exercise, it has some cardiovascular benefits (but not as many as aerobic exercise). With some types of strength training, women have increased their VO_2 max by an average of 8%.

MORE STRENGTH-TRAINING TERMS

Learning the lingo is a necessary but fairly simple evil before you start your exercise program. If you understand what you're doing and why, you'll be able to exercise more effectively and, believe it or not, you'll enjoy it more.

Resistance training is the same thing as strength training. The muscle being exercised must pull against a resistance. The resistance can be a stack of weights on some types of exercise machines or air pressure on other types of machines. The resistance can be a "free weight" (a weight not attached to a machine, such as a dumbbell) that is lifted. There are also resistance exercises that are performed by pulling against a strong, flexible cord that is anchored at one end.

The most common types of equipment used in strength training are free weights or resistance machines. Free weights refers to both dumbbells and barbells. The difference between a dumbbell and a barbell is that the weights can be removed from the bar of the barbell. The dumbbell has a weight that is permanently attached at both ends of the bar.

Resistance machines use an adjustable stack of weights, or air pressure, to provide resistance to lifting. There are a number of major manufacturers of this type of equipment such as Cybex, Nautilus, and Universal.

There are people who advocate the use of machines over the use of free

weights and vice versa for strength-training programs. There are pros and cons for using free weights just as there are for using resistance machines. Some advocates of free weights point out that you can move through a greater range of motion with free weights than you can when using a machine. For other reasons as well, advocates of free weights would say that exercise with these weights more closely approximates the way the muscles are used in real life.

Advocates of resistance machines point out that machines allow you to exert more force throughout the entire movement required by the exercise and therefore exercise more effectively. They also point out that the potential for injury may be less with resistance machines. It is also somewhat more difficult to perform strength-training exercises for the lower body with free weights.

I find that both types of equipment are very useful. Free weights are reasonably inexpensive. If you are going to exercise at home, free weights are practical from the standpoint of expense and space. If you belong to a health club or gym, you will most likely have access to both types of equipment. You can take advantage of the lower body machines and machines for the large back muscles. For variety, if you wish, you can use both free weights and resistance machines.

Reps and sets are important terms as well. Reps is short for repetitions. This is the number of times you perform each exercise at one time. For example, if you lift a dumbbell 8 times in a row, you have just done 8 reps. The term set refers to the completion of each exercise or series of exercises, regardless of how many reps you decided to do. If you repeat exercise A 8 times you have performed 8 reps of exercise A. These 8 reps equal 1 set of exercise

A. On the other hand, if you always do 6 reps of exercise A then 6 reps becomes 1 set of exercise A. A set can also refer to a series of exercises. Let's say you are going to do exercises A, B, C, D, and E. The completion of all five exercises, regardless of how many reps of each you have decided to do, is 1 set.

RM is the abbreviation for repetition maximum. This is a term used in strength training that describes the maximum amount of weight an individual can lift for a specific number of repetitions. For example, if your 1 RM is 50 lbs., that means that you can lift, with good form, 50 lbs. one time only. You could not lift 50 lbs two times and keep good form. Let's say your 6 RM is 20 lbs. That means that you could lift 20 lbs. 6 times in a row and keep good form while lifting. In strength-training programs, a particular RM is usually chosen for each exercise. This is a trial-and-error process at first. You can't know how much weight you can lift for any number of repetitions until you try.

Strictly speaking, a station is a location where a specific exercise is performed. In gyms and health clubs, however, the term station can also mean the exercise itself. When you move from machine to machine, you are said to move from station to station. You could also move to the free weight station, which would be the location where the free weights are kept.

Circuit training and priority training are two different methods of performing sets of resistance-training exercise. Which method you use is determined by your goals in performing strength training. Circuit training emphasizes the development of muscle endurance and cardiovascular benefits. Priority training emphasizes the development of muscular strength. In circuit training, you would perform a greater number of reps at lower weights for each exercise, moving quickly from one exercise or station to the next. You would also do more sets. In priority training, you perform fewer reps using heavier weights for each exercise, taking a brief rest period between each exercise. You would also perform fewer sets. The circuit training method tends to raise the heart rate to a higher level and keep it there, providing a slightly greater cardiovascular benefit than priority training. Priority training, however, has the greater potential for strength increases in the muscles and bone and is preferable for our purposes.

Concentric and eccentric contractions refer to lifting and lowering the weight. It does not matter if you are using free weights or exercise machines. When you lift the weight, a muscle is said to be contracting concentrically. When you lower the weight, the muscle is contracting eccentrically. You can actually lower more weight than you can lift. There are athletes who perform only eccentric strength-training exercises. They do this by having assistants hand them much heavier weights than they could ever lift and then they only have to lower them. While I don't recommend this form of strength training for you, it is useful to understand the difference in the muscles' capabilities during the lifting and lowering phases of strength-training exercise.

ARE YOU READY TO START?

This exercise program combines aerobic and weight-bearing, impact-loading exercises for both the bone and cardiovascular benefits of exercise with priority strength training for the bone and muscle benefits of exercise. These types of exercises are performed on alternate days, 6 days a week. (Everybody needs to rest at least 1 day a week!)

YOUR STRENGTH-TRAINING PROGRAM

Strength-training exercises are designed to exercise specific muscles or groups of muscles. Multiple exercises are needed to completely exercise all of the important muscle groups. In the prevention of osteoporosis, the most important areas are the back, hips and upper legs, and shoulders and arms. That doesn't leave out much, does it?

For each area of the body, exercise machines or free-weight exercises can be used. The choice is really yours, although the resistance machines are easier to use for some types of exercise.

A few important questions must be answered before you begin, such as how many reps and sets you should do and how much weight you should start with. The reps-sets question is a matter of some debate. This issue has been studied by exercise physiologists because they wanted to learn the most effective way to exercise. The lazy side of me wanted to know how little I could do and still get the benefits I needed. Based on the available research for a priority strength-training program, 3 sets of your 6 RM for each exercise are recommended (this is why you have to understand the terminology). This means that you will perform 6 repetitions of each exercise, lifting the maximum amount of weight that you can lift with good form 6 times. After you have completed 6 reps of each exercise, you will repeat all of the exercises 2 more times for a total of 3 sets.

Before you can start, you will have to find out what your 6 RM is for each exercise. That is a matter of trial and error.

If you belong to a club or gym, the trainer should be able to help you by going with you to each station (exercise) and recording the amount of weight that you can lift while he or she observes your form. Make use of these trainers. It is imperative that you understand how to use the equipment properly and safely. You must also know how to adjust the resistance machines to suit your height. The seats are usually adjustable or some other aspect of the machine is adjustable so that most people can be accommodated. Once you know your 6 RM and how to adjust the machines or which dumbbells to use, you are ready to begin.

Other methods can be used in a priority strength-training program. For example, a pyramid system of weight training involves changing the amount of weight lifted every set. In a pyramid system, you might perform 3 sets of each exercise, in which you lift your 6 RM during your first set but lift a lower weight during the second set. In the third set, you would lower the weight even more. You might also prefer to perform 3 sets of your 8 RM (the maximum amount of weight you can lift with good form 8 times, which will be less weight than your 6 RM) instead of 3 sets of your 6 RM. A good weight trainer is a valuable asset in helping you determine the strength-training program that is best for you.

Remember, this is priority strength training. Allow yourself a minute to rest between each exercise. When you lift the weight or, in some cases, push against a weight, this motion is performed fairly quickly. Returning the weight to its original position should be done slowly. In strength-training terminology then, the concentric contraction phase is performed quickly while the eccentric contraction phase is performed slowly.

You also have to breathe while you exercise. It's amazing how many people hold their breath when they perform strength-training exercises. This severely limits the number of reps that you can do! Weight trainers often recommend that you inhale before you start each repetition, holding your breath during the concentric phase of the exercise, and exhale during the eccentric phase or at the completion of the rep. Other experts have recommended that you exhale during the lift and inhale while lowering the weight. I prefer the second approach because I find it more natural and it prevents undesirable increases in chest and abdominal pressure during the lifting phase. The most important aspect of breathing during strength training is *to keep breathing*. It's more important to breathe regularly than to worry about inhaling or exhaling at a specific time.

EXERCISES FOR THE BACK

The back extension. If you have access to a back-extension resistance machine, take advantage of it. This is one of the most effective and easiest ways to exercise the back extensors, the large muscles that run up and down either side of the spine. You sit on a saddle leaning back against a padded bar that comes across the back just below the shoulder blades. During the exercise, you push back against the bar, raising the stack of weights.

To perform back-extension exercises without a back-extension machine is somewhat difficult. One way is by doing a floor exercise in which you raise the head and shoulders off the floor while lying face down. This exercise is more difficult if you lift your feet from the floor at the same time you lift your head and shoulders. Weights can also be used in this exercise. Weighted discs, wrapped in a towel, can be held on the back of the head or placed on the back by a partner during the lift. This is rather difficult to do, however.

EXERCISES FOR THE SHOULDERS, UPPER ARMS, UPPER AND MIDDLE BACK

The lat pull-down. In this exercise, you sit underneath a bar and grasp it with an overhand grip. Your hands should be placed on the bar farther apart than the width of your shoulders. Sitting up straight, you pull the bar down behind

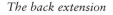

The back extension

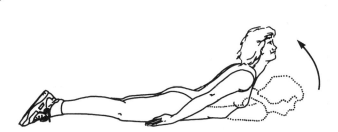

The floor back extension

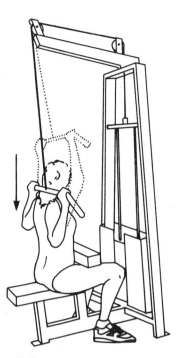

The lat pull-down

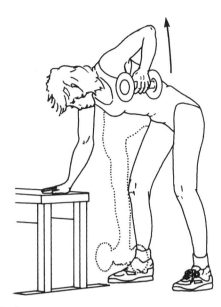

The bent-over row

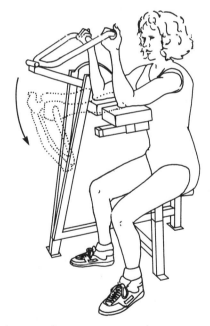

The bicep curl

your head or in front of your head to chest level. If you pull the bar down in front, the muscles in the upper chest are worked harder than when the bar is pulled down behind the head. The lat pull-down strengthens the large back muscles and the muscles of the upper chest and arms.

The bent-over row is a free-weight exercise that essentially works the same muscles as the behind-the-head lat pull-down. Place your feet comfortably apart. When you bend from the waist, keep your back straight or even slightly arched; do not round your back. Lift the weight straight up, resulting in the bent elbow being lifted above the back. Keep the knees slightly bent during the exercise.

EXERCISES FOR THE UPPER ARM

The bicep curl. This exercise can be done using a resistance machine or with free weights. While seated with your feet placed comfortably apart, rest your elbows on the shoulder-level pad. Using an underhand grip, grasp the handles and pull them toward your shoulders.

Bicep curls are easy to do with free weights. Standing with your feet comfortably apart, grasp a dumbbell or small barbell in each hand. Your elbows should be slightly in front of and against your body. The palms face outward. Lift the weight, alternating each arm. Bring the weight up more quickly than you lower it. To use strength-training terms, the concentric muscle contraction should be performed more quickly than the eccentric contraction. Having your elbows against your body protects you from hyperextending your elbow during the exercise. It also helps keep you from cheating by using your shoulder muscles to help lift the weight.

The tricep extension. The tricep is the muscle on the back of the upper arm. It is usually the weaker of the two muscles in the upper arm. This is also the area of the arm that, quite frankly, is so often flabby in women. To use the resistance machine for this exercise, you begin much like you do for the bicep curl machine: sit with your feet positioned comfortably apart and your back straight. Rest your elbows on a padded shelf, just below shoulder height. Grasp both levers by the handles

and pull them down, until forearms are parallel to the floor.

This exercise can also be done with free weights. Grasp a dumbbell or barbell with both hands and hold it behind your head. Try to keep your arms close to your head, elbows pointing up. Begin the exercise with the weight hanging down behind your head. Raise the weight by straightening your arms. The arms should not make any other type of movement. Lower the weight carefully and slowly. Again the concentric phase should be faster than the eccentric phase. Don't hit yourself in the back with the weight when you lower it!

EXERCISES FOR THE LOWER ARM OR FOREARM

The wrist curl. This exercise is best performed with free weights, although machines can be used as well. To use the free weights, sit on a weight bench (a chair will also do). Holding the weight in the arm to be exercised, lay the back of your arm down on your thigh. Your arm must be flat on your thigh from the elbow to the wrist. The palm of your hand, holding the weight,

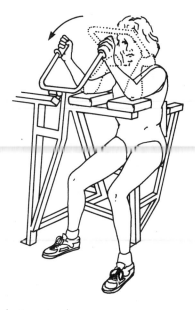

The triceps extension

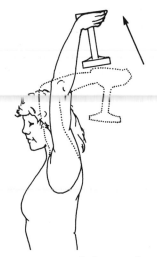

The triceps extension with free weights

should be face up. Allow your hand to drop down over the knee. Now raise or curl the hand up and then lower it back down. After completing your reps with one hand, repeat using the other hand.

The wrist extension. This is the opposite of the wrist curl. It exercises the muscles on the back of the forearm. This exercise is also performed seated, holding the dumbbell in the hand to be exercised. Just as in the wrist curl, lay your arm, from the elbow to the wrist, down on your thigh, allowing your hand to hang over your knee. Now roll your arm over so that the palm of your hand is facing toward the floor. To perform the exercise raise the hand up and then lower the weight back down.

For both the wrist curl and the wrist extension you will find that you must bend forward from the waist in order to lay your forearm down on your thigh. When you do, bend forward with a slight arch in your back. Do not round your back forward.

EXERCISES FOR THE HIP, UPPER AND LOWER LEGS

The leg press. Using a resistance machine, you begin this exercise with your knees

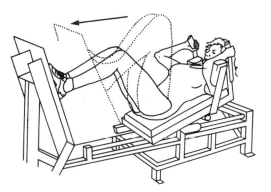

The leg press

pulled up toward your chest. You then push against the foot rest using the muscles of the buttocks, thighs, and lower legs. You should not completely straighten your legs during the push. There should be a very slight bend in the knee at the end of the push or concentric contraction phase.

The only free-weight exercise that simulates the leg press is called the lunge. This exercise also requires total body balance and coordination and that you have no knee problems. For the dumbbell lunge, dumbbells are held in each hand at your sides. Step forward on either foot, allowing your body to slowly sink down as low as you can go. You must keep your back

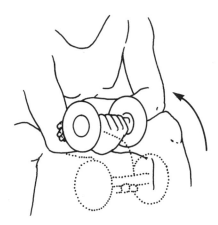

The wrist curl with free weights

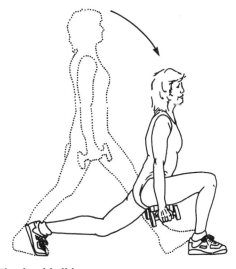

The dumbbell lunge

straight. You then come back up and step backward to your original starting position. You can judge the distance you should step forward by noting if your knee is over your foot (correct positioning) when you are at the lowest part of your lunge.

In the barbell lunge, a barbell is held behind the head on the shoulders. The movements are otherwise the same. This is an excellent exercise for total body coordination and balance as well as for various muscles. Having tried it myself, I must confess I prefer the leg press machine. It's really embarrassing if you can't get back up after the lunge!

The quadriceps extension. The quadriceps are the large muscles on the front of the upper leg. They straighten the leg at the knee joint. The knee-extension machine is the resistance machine for this exercise. The exercise is begun with the feet hooked behind a padded bar. Your legs should actually be a little behind you, but not so much that it hurts. If it does, you probably need to add some padding to the back rest so that you can sit farther forward on the machine. Both legs are then straightened simultaneously. Don't pop your legs up and don't lock your

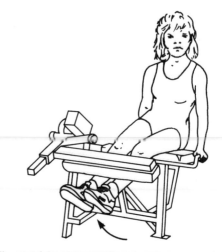

The quadriceps extension

knees at the end of the contraction (the concentric phase, remember?). Then slowly and deliberately lower the bar but don't allow your legs to return to the original position completely until you have finished your last repetition.

To perform a quadriceps extension with free weights, you need a weighted boot. This is a device that you can attach a weight to and fit over your shoes. Normally, one leg is exercised at a time, rather than both legs as is done with the machine. The best way to use the boot is to sit on a padded weight bench so that the end of the bench is against the back of your knee. Place your hands on the sides of the bench and keep your back straight during the exercise. The leg is then straightened and lowered for the chosen number of repetitions (this would be 6, using your 6 RM).

The knee curl. The muscles in the back of the thigh are called the hamstrings. The hamstrings bend the knee. They can be exercised with both resistance machines or a free-weight boot. You lie face down with a padded bar across the back of your ankles. Ideally, your kneecaps should be just over the edge of the bench. The legs are then bent at the knees, raising the bar up

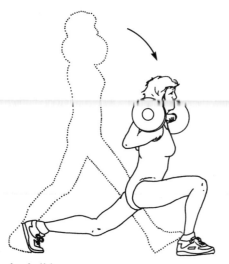

The barbell lunge

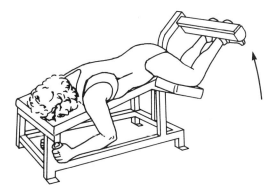

The knee curl

against the chosen weight. It is important to lower the bar down slowly during the eccentric contraction phase to avoid hurting your knees.

The knee curl can also be done using the free-weight boot. This exercise is usually performed standing. You do need to hold on to a support during this exercise. Keep your back straight and head up. Now, lift the weighted boot by bending

your leg at the knee and pulling it up toward your hip. Lower your leg to the ground slowly. Only one leg at a time is exercised when using the boot.

The calf raise. The calf muscles in the lower legs can be easily strengthened by using free weights, although there are machines designed for this purpose as well. To use the free weights, simply hold the chosen amount of weight in each hand with your arms at your sides. Your palms should be facing your sides. With your feet placed 6 to 8 inches apart, raise up on your toes and then lower your heels back to the floor. Do not pull your shoulders up during this exercise. Your arms should hang at your sides.

The shoulder shrug. The calf raise can be altered slightly for your shoulders. Again, holding a weight in each hand with your arms at your sides, palms facing your sides, shrug both shoulders up as high as they will go. Then lower them back down to the original position.

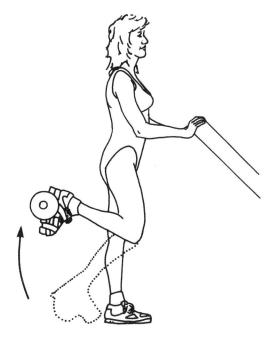

The knee curl with weighted boot

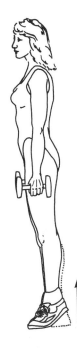

The calf raise

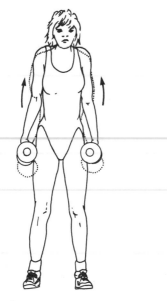

The shoulder shrug

There are many other machines and free-weight exercises you can do, but these exercises are the most important for strength training as part of your osteoporosis-prevention regimen. Three days a week seems to be an effective schedule for strength training. Most authorities recommend at least 3 days a week with no more than 2 "off" days in a row.

YOUR AEROBIC, WEIGHT-BEARING EXERCISE PROGRAM

Brisk walking or jogging is the simplest and most effective weight-bearing, impact-loading exercise for an osteoporosis-prevention exercise program. When I discuss this aspect of the exercise program with my patients, they often comment that they are on their feet all day long anyway. Doesn't that count as weight-bearing exercise? Of course, it counts for something. It's just that the impact loading of the bones during standing and casual walking is not sufficient to stimulate the bones or heart. Obtaining the recommended cardio-

vascular benefits and bone benefits requires a little more effort.

Regardless of your age, a walking or jogging program must progress gradually. If you are unable to walk at a pace of 4 mph for 50 minutes, you certainly can't jog at a pace of 6 or 7 mph for 50 minutes. The minimum goal of this phase of the exercise program is a 5 mph walk for 50 minutes. That means that you can walk 1 mile in 12 minutes. I know that I can walk at a 4 mph pace and I can jog at a 6 mph pace, but I can't walk at a 5 mph pace. I am only about 5'1" and, quite frankly, it's more comfortable for my short legs to jog at 6 mph than to try to walk at 5 mph. You may be able to walk at a 5 mph pace without difficulty. This is your minimum goal, however, so feel free to exceed 5 mph in speed as long as you work up to it gradually.

Before you begin, you will need to decide where you are going to walk or jog. Did you ever wonder why people jog in the street instead of on the sidewalk? These people really aren't suicidal. They are trying to protect their joints from injury. Many streets will have a coating of some type over the cement that provides some cushioning for runners. Most sidewalks don't. If you have access to a track of some kind—whether it is dirt, grass, or a special cushioned surface—try to use it. Your feet and knees will thank you.

Your feet will also be grateful if you have the proper shoes. Casual shoes with rubber soles were not intended to protect your feet during brisk walking or jogging. Walking and running shoes are specially designed to provide your feet with the stability and protection they need during walking or running. Other types of athletic shoes, although they may be excellent for the activity for which they were designed, should not be used for brisk walking or jogging. Tennis shoes, for example (real tennis shoes made for playing tennis) are intended to support the foot during the side-to-side motion required by tennis, not the front-to-back motion of the foot that occurs during walking or running. Tennis shoes also have extra protection for the ball of the foot, while running shoes tend to protect the heel. You don't have to spend a fortune for good shoes, but they are a necessity.

Your first time out on the track (or wherever you have decided to exercise) you need to find out what you can do now. You will need a watch and some means of determining how far you have walked or jogged. Many tracks post a notice indicating the number of laps that constitute a mile. If you are walking in your neighborhood, you can measure the distance with the odometer in your car by driving the same distance you walk. The first time, I want you to walk or jog at a comfortable pace for as long as you can up to a maximum of 50 minutes. Once you have settled into the pace you will continue to exercise at, take your pulse (in your wrist) for 10 seconds and remember this number. When you find that you must slow down to the point that you consider to be a normal, casual pace in order to continue, you have reached your stopping point for this first venture. Note your distance and the time you exercised. Now calculate your average speed by dividing the distance by the time. For example, if you covered 2 miles in 30 minutes you averaged a pace of 4 miles per hour. The actual calculation is: 2 miles ÷ 0.5 hour = 4 mph.

If you found that you could maintain a pace of 5 mph or greater but you simply could not keep going the whole 50 minutes, then you will need to concentrate primarily on your endurance. On the other hand, if you were able to exercise the entire 50 minutes but only averaged a pace of 3 mph, you will need to concentrate on

improving your speed. Most of us need to work on both aspects of this part of the program, but one area may need more work than the other.

Remember your pulse, which you counted for 10 seconds? Multiply this number by 6. This is your heart rate in beats per minute for your initial level of exercise. Calculate your maximum heart rate and compare this to the one you measured while exercising. (Your maximum heart rate is 220 minus your age. If you are 45, then your maximum heart rate is 220 − 45, or 175. If you are 65, then your maximum heart rate is 220 − 65, or 155.) To obtain significant cardiovascular benefits from this exercise, you would like to have your heart rate between 70% and 90% of your maximum heart rate. For the 45-year-old, that would be a heart rate between 123 and 158. For the 65-year-old, this would be a heart rate between 109 and 140.

Even though getting your heart rate into the target heart range is desirable for cardiovascular benefits from this exercise, if you are over 50 you must proceed with caution. If you find that during your initial exercise session, your heart rate exceeds 60% of your maximum heart rate, you must see your doctor before beginning this exercise program. For the 65-year-old woman, a heart rate greater than 93 beats per minute during her initial session requires that she obtain clearance from her doctor before proceeding with the program. Other medical considerations are discussed in chapter 6.

THE ENDURANCE PROGRAM

Because your minimum goal is a pace of 5 mph for 50 minutes, you should ultimately be able to cover a minimum distance of 4.2 miles in 50 minutes (5 mph × 50 min ÷ 60 min = 4.2 miles). You will need to know how many laps or how many times around the block constitute 4.2 miles in order to follow this program. Over a period of several weeks, gradually increase the distance that you briskly walk or jog while maintaining the same speed. Don't be tempted to jump ahead. The gradual increases in distance allow you to progress safely in the exercise program.

To illustrate how the endurance program works, let's say that you were able to walk briskly at a pace of 5 mph, but had to stop after 30 minutes. Your goal is a total time of 50 minutes. The program will call for you to increase your time walked by 5 minutes each week.

Notice that during your first full week you should not attempt to increase your total time from your baseline value. Once you have reached your elapsed time goal of 50 minutes, you can continue to increase your speed if you wish but you do not have to increase your total time beyond 50 minutes for this program. Remember, you will be performing your aerobic, weight-bearing exercise 3 days a week, on alternate days. The goal for that week, that is, the increase in time by a total of 5 minutes from the previous week, need only be reached by the last aerobic exercise day of the week. You will obviously need to keep a record of your progress. A sim-

ple note pad will do, although a runner's diary, available from any athletic or running shoe store, is designed for this type of record keeping. If you are unable to meet the elapsed time goal by the third aerobic exercise day, stay at that level for an additional week before attempting additional increases in elapsed time.

THE SPEED PROGRAM

The speed program is similar to the endurance program in that we will start with your baseline values and progress gradually. You will always walk 50 minutes during your aerobic, weight-bearing exercise sessions but you will increase your speed each week. To illustrate the basic principles of the speed program, let's say that you walked 50 minutes but you only averaged a pace of 3 mph. Your minimum goal is a pace of 5 mph.

Notice that during the first full week of exercise, you should not attempt to increase your speed from your baseline values. Your distance will also remain the same. The speed and distance goals for each subsequent week need only be

SAMPLE ENDURANCE PROGRAM			
	Speed	Elapsed Time	Distance
Baseline	5 mph	30 minutes	2.5 miles
Week 1	5 mph	30 minutes	2.5 miles
Week 2	5 mph	35 minutes	2.9 miles
Week 3	5 mph	40 minutes	3.3 miles
Week 4	5 mph	45 minutes	3.8 miles
Week 5	5 mph	50 minutes	4.2 miles

SAMPLE SPEED PROGRAM			
	Speed	Elapsed Time	Distance
Baseline	3 mph	50 minutes	2.5 miles
Week 1	3 mph	50 minutes	2.5 miles
Week 2	3.5 mph	50 minutes	2.9 miles
Week 3	3.5 mph	50 minutes	2.9 miles
Week 4	4 mph	50 minutes	3.3 miles
Week 5	4 mph	50 minutes	3.3 miles
Week 6	4.5 mph	50 minutes	3.8 miles
Week 7	4.5 mph	50 minutes	3.8 miles
Week 8	5 mph	50 minutes	4.2 miles

reached by the last day of the exercise week for that speed and distance level. While you should expect to feel tired when you complete your 50 minutes of exercise, you should not feel bad. If you do, then the level of exercise is too strenuous. You need to drop back a level and progress more slowly.

THE COMBINATION SPEED-ENDURANCE PROGRAM

Some of us cannot keep up a pace of 5 mph for any length of time and cannot walk briskly for 50 minutes without stopping. The combination speed-endurance program is most appropriate here.

SAMPLE COMBINATION SPEED-ENDURANCE PROGRAM FOR FIRST 4 WEEKS

	Speed	Elapsed Time	Distance
Baseline	2.6 mph	35 minutes	1.5 miles
Week 1	2.6 mph	35 minutes	1.5 miles
Week 2			
Day 1	3.1 mph	35 minutes	1.8 miles
Days 2 & 3	2.6 mph	40 minutes	1.7 miles
Week 3			
Day 1	3.1 mph	35 minutes	1.8 miles
Days 2 & 3	2.6 mph	45 minutes	2.0 miles
Week 4			
Day 1	3.6 mph	35 minutes	2.1 miles
Days 2 & 3	2.6 mph	50 minutes	2.2 miles

SAMPLE COMBINATION SPEED-ENDURANCE PROGRAM—WEEKS 5–8

	Speed	Elapsed Time	Distance
Week 5			
Day 1	3.6 mph	35 minutes	2.1 miles
Days 2 & 3	2.6 mph	50 minutes	2.2 miles
Week 6			
Day 1	3.6 mph	40 minutes	2.4 miles
Days 2 & 3	3.1 mph	50 minutes	2.6 miles
Week 7			
Day 1	3.6 mph	45 minutes	2.7 miles
Days 2 & 3	3.1 mph	50 minutes	2.6 miles
Week 8			
Day 1	3.6 mph	50 minutes	3.0 miles
Days 2 & 3	3.6 mph	50 minutes	3.0 miles

To illustrate this program, let's say that you walked as briskly as you could for 35 minutes but then found yourself slowing down. You had covered a distance of 1.5 miles, which according to your calculations meant that you had kept up a pace of 2.6 mph before stopping. (The calculation to determine your pace is as follows: distance divided by time equals speed or 1.5 miles divided by 0.58 hours equals 2.6 mph; 35 minutes divided by 60 minutes equals 0.58 hours.) With these baseline values, both the speed and endurance are only about half as good as we need for the bones and heart to benefit from the exercise. In the combination speed-endurance program we will gradually increase both.

For the first week of the program, you should not attempt to increase either your total time or speed from your baseline values. In the second week and the weeks that follow, 2 of the 3 days are devoted to increasing your endurance and 1 day is devoted to increasing your speed.

The first week of the combination program there is no attempt to increase the time walked or the speed walked from the original baseline values. From the second week on, the speed with which you walk is increased on day 1 by 0.5 mph every two weeks. Every week, on days 2 and 3, the total time walked is increased by 5 minutes from the previous week although there should be no deliberate attempt to walk any faster than you did originally. You will find that you do walk faster simply because you are becoming more fit, but you should not deliberately attempt to walk faster on these days. As you can see, in this sample program, the endurance goal of 50 minutes was reached by week 4. It will take several more weeks to reach the speed goal.

The endurance time goal of 50 minutes was reached during week 4 on days 2 and 3. We had been concentrating on speed only on day 1 during the first 4 weeks. While the speed had improved, the goal of 5 mph had not been reached. During weeks 5 through 8, we have reversed the emphasis of day 1 and days 2 and 3. Day 1 has now become an endurance day and the emphasis for days 2 and 3 is on improving speed. On day 1 every week during weeks 5 through 8, the total time walked is increased by 5 minutes until the goal of 50 minutes is reached by week 8. In the meantime, every 2 weeks the speed walked on days 2 and 3 is increased by 0.5 mph. By week 8 of the program, the values for speed, time, and distance are the same for all 3 days. Keeping the total time walked at 50 minutes on all three days from here on and increasing the speed walked by 0.5 mph every other week, it will take an additional 6 weeks to reach the goal of a 50-minute brisk walk or slow jog at 5 mph.

In the last 6 weeks, the same routine is followed on all 3 days. What began as the combination speed-endurance program evolves into the speed program only.

SAMPLE SPEED-ENDURANCE PROGRAM— WEEKS 9–14			
	Speed	Elapsed Time	Distance
Week 9	3.6 mph	50 minutes	3.0 miles
Week 10	4.1 mph	50 minutes	3.4 miles
Week 11	4.1 mph	50 minutes	3.4 miles
Week 12	4.6 mph	50 minutes	3.8 miles
Week 13	4.6 mph	50 minutes	3.8 miles
Week 14	5.1 mph	50 minutes	4.2 miles

In setting up and following your own program, it's imperative that you have some way of knowing how far you have walked or jogged. Since none of us have built-in speedometers, the only way we can know if we have walked at a certain speed is to reach a set distance by the allotted time. For example, in week 10, the only way that I could know if I had walked at a speed of 4.1 mph is to have covered a distance of 3.4 miles in 50 minutes. I must be able to calculate how many laps around the track or times around the block equals this distance to know if I have met my goal. This isn't as difficult as it may sound but it does require some planning.

Phillip Walker, M.S.S., an exercise physiologist and consultant at the Cooper Clinic, developed the concept of a speed, endurance, and combination program. For all three programs, the basic guidelines are the same.

One Last Pep Talk

You can do this. It's 1 hour a day, 6 days a week to keep your heart, bones, and muscles fit and healthy. That's only 6 hours a week out of the entire 168 hours in a week. Anyone who exercises regularly will confirm that you will be far more productive for the remaining 162 hours in the week because you will feel better, have more energy, be stronger, and have a brighter mental outlook as a result of the time you devoted to exercise.

I really do understand what I'm asking you to do. I work full time and have home and family responsibilities. I also travel a great deal. I know (and have used) every excuse in the book not to exercise. There are times when circumstances beyond my control force me to abandon my regular exercise routine. There are other times when the spirit is willing but the body isn't. But I know what osteoporosis can do to a woman. I know that it can destroy the quality of my life. It can take away my independence. It can leave me with pain while it alters my appearance. Osteoporosis can even kill me. So I get out of the office, out of the kitchen, or off the couch and back to my exercise program.

BASIC GUIDELINES FOR SPEED, ENDURANCE, AND COMBINATION SPEED-ENDURANCE PROGRAMS

1. Establish your baseline values for total time and distance.
2. Reaching the endurance goal is more important initially than meeting the speed goal.
3. Do not increase your speed more than 0.5 mph every 2 weeks.
4. Do not increase your total time more than 5 minutes every week.
5. If you feel ill after or during exercise, stop. Drop your speed and elapsed time values back to the previous week.
6. Keep a record of your progress.
7. If you are over 50 and your heart rate exceeds 60% of your maximum heart rate during your baseline session, see your doctor before beginning the exercise program.

CHAPTER 8

Exercise for the Woman with Osteoporosis

Exercise is an extraordinarily important part of any osteoporosis prevention or treatment program. The woman who already has osteoporosis must approach her exercise program differently than the woman who is exercising to prevent osteoporosis. We discussed the definition of osteoporosis earlier, but remember that you are considered to have osteoporosis if you have lost sufficient bone to be at risk for having a fracture. You need not have already had a fracture. You must recognize that certain exercises might actually increase your risk of having a fracture and must be avoided.

Improving muscular strength, even without improving bone strength, is a desirable goal in order to improve individuals' abilities to rise from a chair or stop themselves from falling. Exercises designed to improve balance and flexibility also assume added importance for this group of women. In general, because women who are exercising as part of the treatment of osteoporosis tend to be older than women who are exercising to prevent osteoporosis, the intensity or difficulty of the exercises is less initially and progresses more slowly for overall safety.

A woman who has had an osteoporotic fracture may be in too much pain to perform some types of exercise. If you have had a spinal fracture that has occurred in the last 6 months, it may still cause pain and prevent you from performing some of the exercises recommended here. You will simply have to go a little slower than a woman who may be at risk for fracture but has not yet had one. Nevertheless, it is desirable for you to start exercising as soon as your pain will permit. Bone loss, which only increases your risk of having an additional fracture, is accelerated by inactivity and prolonged bed rest. If you have had a hip fracture, you must discuss any proposed exercise program with your doctor first. Depending on the type of hip fracture you had, the treatment that followed, and the length of time since it occurred, some exercises may be unsuitable or even dangerous for you to do.

THE BASIC SAFETY RULES

The cardinal rule is to talk with your doctor about any exercise program before beginning. The doctor who has had the privilege of caring for you will know your medical history in great detail. This knowledge will allow him or her to judge the safety and benefit of any exercise program for you as an individual. Your doctor may suggest changes in an exercise program I would recommend because he or she has a personal knowledge of your medical history.

I have no doubt whatsoever that exercise is extremely beneficial for the woman who has osteoporosis, regardless of her age. But before you begin your exercise program, I want to be sure that you exercise safely. For women with osteoporosis, both those who have had a fracture and those who are only at increased risk of having a fracture, there are four important safety rules you must follow.

THE FOUR EXERCISE DON'TS FOR THE WOMAN WITH OSTEOPOROSIS

1. DON'T perform any exercise or activity that jars the spine. In medical terms, this would be called impact loading of the spine. This type of activity increases the risk of spinal fracture because the weakened vertebrae cannot tolerate this force. This means no jumping, no high-impact aerobics, no jogging or running. (I do recommend impact-loading exercises for preventing osteoporosis, but not for the woman who already has osteoporosis.)

2. DON'T perform any exercise or activity that requires you to bend forward from the waist with the back rounded. The medical term for this posture is spinal flexion. This dramatically increases the forces on your spine, increasing the danger of a collapsed vertebra. This means no sit-ups, no toe-touches, no "crunches" (an exercise term for popular abdominal-muscle exercises), no rowing machines that require this position.

3. DON'T perform any exercise or activity that makes falls likely. That means no trampolines or step aerobics. Don't exercise on slippery floors (including wooden gym floors, where droplets of sweat might accumulate) or in hard,

smooth-soled shoes. Don't even go to the gym or club when the sidewalks are icy!

4. DON'T perform any exercise or activity that requires you to move your leg sideways or across your body against resistance. The medical term for this movement is abduction and adduction of the leg. This will generally only apply to certain types of resistance-exercise machines. A weakened hip may be more susceptible to breaking when stressed in this manner.

These DON'Ts are outlined for your safety and must be followed. As long as you eliminate the DON'Ts, there is every expectation that you can exercise safely. So what should you DO?

THE FOUR EXERCISE DO'S FOR THE WOMAN WITH OSTEOPOROSIS

1. DO follow a regular walking program (with your ultimate goal being a minimum pace of 3 mph for 50 minutes 5 days a week. This appears to be the minimum speed and time necessary to maintain the bones' strength. Walking at 3 mph on level ground uses 3 METS of expended energy. A 4 mph walk will use 4.2 METS. This will have some benefit for your heart and lungs. Improvement in endurance and agility will also lessen the likelihood of falling.

2. DO strength-training exercises. You can lift weights. It is not unfeminine and can be done safely. This can be free weights (the little dumbbells) or resistance-exercise machines. Special emphasis should be placed on exercises for the hip, thighs, back, arms, and shoulders.

3. DO exercises to improve balance and agility.

4. DO spine-extension exercises. This is the opposite of spinal flexion, which must be avoided. (See DON'T rule #2). Spine-extension exercises are performed by arching the back and are quite safe. These exercises can be done sitting in a chair with or without any resistance to the basic motion of arching the back. These exercises strengthen the back extensor muscles, the large muscles that hold the spine erect, reducing the development of a dowager's hump, reducing back fatigue, and strengthening the spine itself.

GETTING STARTED

To borrow an old saying, Rome wasn't built in a day. An exercise program for osteoporosis is like Rome. You must start gradually in order to avoid injury and allow your body to build endurance and strength over a period of time. As a consequence, the types of exercises you do initially, and the effort they require, will not be as strenuous as they will later on. Don't be tempted to go too fast or to skip ahead. Doing so would only create the potential for injury.

The exercise program consists of a balance between the aerobic weight-bearing activity of walking, isotonic strength training to target the areas of the skeleton where fractures occur and to improve coordination and balance, isometric abdominal exercises, and spine-extension exercises.

BACK-EXTENSION EXERCISES AND ISOMETRIC ABDOMINAL EXERCISES

These exercises were designed specifically for the woman with osteoporosis by Dr. Mehrsheed Sinaki and her colleagues at the Mayo Clinic. They are excellent exercises, even for the woman who is still limited somewhat by pain from a recent spinal fracture. These exercises do not cause an increase in pain. In fact, most of my patients tell me the exercises actually make them feel better. The exercises are also very safe, even for a fragile spine.

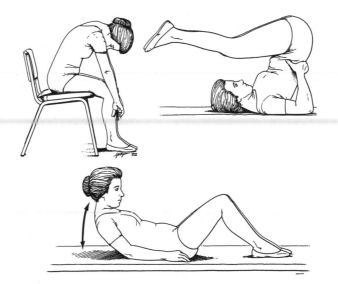

Exercises to avoid. ©1985 the Mayo Foundation

Back extension is safe because the spine is capable of withstanding a great deal of force as long as it is straight or slightly arched.

The benefits of back-extension exercises are a reduction in pain and an increase in the strength of the muscles that support the spine. Strengthening the back muscles has other benefits as well. Because these muscles are responsible for holding us erect, strengthening the back extensor muscles helps counteract the tendency to become stooped. Back fatigue and weakness are reduced. Because some of these muscles attach to the spine itself, the exercises also act as a mild strengthening stimulus to the spine.

The abdominal or stomach muscles also help to support the back. Many familiar exercises for the stomach muscles involve trunk flexion, which a woman with osteoporosis should avoid. Sit-ups are a perfect example of an exercise for the stomach muscles that requires you to bend forward from the waist with the back rounded. A sit-up is nothing more than touching your toes while lying down instead of standing up. Both activities involve trunk flexion. So how can we strengthen the stomach muscles without using trunk flexion? We can use isometric abdominal exercises to effectively strengthen the stomach muscles without placing any strain on the spine and increasing the risk of fracture.

The first two back-extension exercises are "chair" extension exercises. They can also be done just as effectively while standing. If you use a chair, the chair should have a low back and no arms in order to allow you to perform the exercise properly. To begin chair extension exercise number 1, sit away from the back of the chair. Remember to sit up tall and keep your chin up. Raise your arms and place your hands on the back of your head. You may rest your fingers against the back of your head or lock your hands across the back of your head. If you lock your hands, be sure *not* to pull on your neck. Now, gently and slowly, but firmly, push your elbows back as far as they will go. Do not jerk the elbows back, do not perform this motion quickly. Once your elbows are as far back as they will go, let them come forward and relax. Repeat this exercise 10 times. Check to be sure that you are sitting up straight with your chin up as you

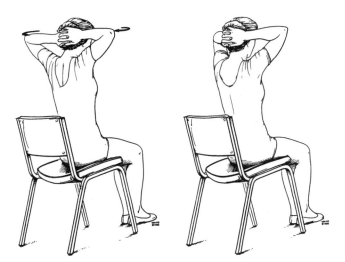

Sinaki chair extension exercise no. 1. ©1985 the Mayo Foundation

perform the repetitions. If you cannot perform 10 initially, start with 5 and increase this number by at least 1 every week. Repeat this exercise twice a day, every day.

After you have finished extension exercise number 1, simply drop your arms down by your side for number 2. Bend the arms at the elbow, keeping your hands relaxed. Again, remember to sit up straight. The motion used during this exercise is the same motion you would use if you were trying to touch your elbows behind your back. You can't do this of course. It's just the motion I want you to imitate. With your arms bent, take your elbows back, gently and slowly. Do not jerk them back! When you have taken them as far back as they will go, let them come forward and relax. While you are performing this exercise, check to be sure that you are sitting up straight with your chin up as before. Also check to see that your shoulders are remaining relaxed. People have a tendency to lift their shoulders with each repetition until the shoulders are held so high that the arms really can't move. Like chair extension exercise number 1, repeat this exercise 10 times. If necessary, start with 5 and work your way

up to 10 by increasing the number of repetitions by at least 1 each week. Do this exercise twice a day, every day. These chair extension exercises strengthen the extensor muscles of the upper back.

The next back-extension exercise is a floor exercise. You must be able to get down on the floor to perform this exercise. If you are recovering from a recent fracture and cannot get up and down from the floor just yet, you must wait to add this exercise to your routine.

To perform this exercise, which I call a floor leg lift, get down on your hands and knees on the floor. (If you have hardwood floors or want extra cushioning, use an exercise mat.) Lift your left leg, with the knee bent, as high as you can slowly and smoothly. Then lower the leg to the floor, coming to rest again on your knee. Do not jerk the leg up. Remember to keep the knee bent. The leg should not be straight as it is lifted. You should lift each leg 10 times if possible. You can alternate legs, that is, lift first one and then the other or you can lift one leg 10 times and then the other leg 10 times. The major consideration that determines how you do this is the comfort of your knees. If you cannot lift each leg at least 10 times, begin with 5 and work your way up, increasing the number of lifts for each leg by at least 1 a week. The floor leg-lift extension exercise should also be done twice a day, every day.

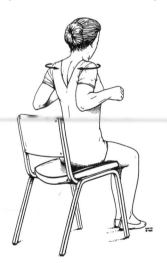

Sinaki chair extension exercise no. 2. ©1985 the Mayo Foundation

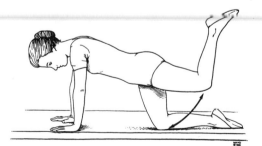

Sinaki leg-lift back extension. ©1985 the Mayo Foundation

This exercise strengthens the extensor muscles of the lower spine and the hip.

The next two exercises are isometric abdominal exercises to strengthen the stomach muscles that help support the back. X rays have actually been taken of women while they were performing these exercises in order to prove that these isometric abdominal exercises do not cause the spine to flex or curve forward when done properly. Remember, I want you to avoid flexion because this might increase your risk of having a spinal fracture. Much like the floor leg lift, you should be able to get down on the floor to perform these exercises. If your mattress is very firm, you may be able to perform these while lying in bed.

The first isometric abdominal exercise is often called a modified sit-up. Lie on the floor (or bed) with your knees bent and place your arms down at your sides. Begin this exercise with your head on the floor. Lift your head only far enough so that your shoulders begin to lift from the floor. Now stop. That is far enough. Lower your head to the floor. As in every other exercise that we have discussed, the lift should be gentle. Do not jerk your head up. Perform the exercise slowly. Speed actually detracts from the benefit of the exercise. Repeat 10 times twice a day,

every day. If you cannot initially perform 10 repetitions, reduce the initial number to 5 as before, increasing the number every week as your strength improves.

If you have some arthritis in your neck and lifting your head in this manner causes neck pain, this exercise can be modified in the following manner. Again, lie flat on the floor with the knees bent. Allow your head to remain on the floor. (You can put a pillow under your head if you like.) Place your hands on your abdomen. Now, without moving your head or any other part of your body, tighten, or suck in, your stomach muscles and hold this position for a count of 3. You should feel your stomach muscles get hard under your hands. After a count of 3, relax. Take two or three breaths before repeating this exercise. Repeat the exercise 10 times if possible. If not, do 5 and work your way up. Perform the exercise twice a day, every day.

For the second isometric abdominal exercise, lie on a flat, firm surface to begin. (The surface must be extremely firm in order to perform this exercise properly.) Slip your hands under your hips. Do not raise your head during the exercise. Now lift your feet off the floor, keeping your

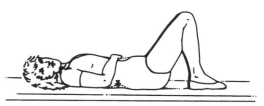

Isometric abdominal exercise

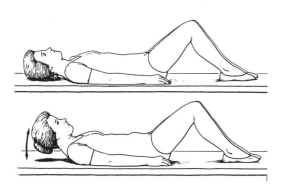

Sinaki isometric abdominal exercise. ©1985 the Mayo Foundation

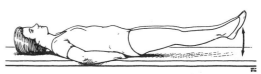

Sinaki isometric abdominal leg lift. ©1985 the Mayo Foundation

legs straight. Your feet should come off the floor about 6 inches. Lower your feet back to the floor. Again, do not jerk your feet up and do not try to perform this exercise quickly. This is perhaps the most difficult of all the exercises described so far. Don't be discouraged if you find that you cannot perform more than 3 or 4 of these before tiring. Your goal will be 10 repetitions. Do what you can at first, gradually working your way up to 10. This exercise, like the others, should be done twice a day, every day.

The last exercise I want you to do is not for the back or stomach but for your legs. Specifically, it is for your thighs, to strengthen the muscles that help you get out of a chair or squat to pick up something off the floor. In fact, I call this exercise a half squat. You need to hold on to something approximately waist high, like a heavy piece of furniture or railing while performing the half squat. Whatever you use, it must be anchored in place or so heavy that it could not possibly move. Stand with your feet comfortably apart. Stand up straight. While holding on to the object you've chosen, lower your body by bending your knees. Go only about half-

way down. Do not do a complete knee bend. Go down slowly and gently. Now, come back up. Repeat the half squat 15 times if possible. As you perform this exercise, remember to keep your back straight and your chin up. Perform this exercise twice a day, every day.

These six exercises take very little time to do. Even performing all six twice a day takes 30 minutes at most. These exercises, combined with the walking program, form the basis of the osteoporosis exercise program. As you become stronger, it will be time to advance your exercise program and "pump a little iron."

THE WALKING PROGRAM

It really doesn't matter where you walk. You can walk inside in a mall, outside on the sidewalk or park path, on a track, or on a treadmill. The setting is really determined by what's convenient, what's enjoyable, and what's safe. Safety refers not only to crime-related concerns but also to the surface you walk on. The surface should be smooth and provide good traction. A flat surface is fine. You don't need to be climbing hills. Treadmills work as well as tracks for walking, but you must be sure you know how to get on and off them. We've all seen the comedy routines in which an individual goes flying off the back of a treadmill or falls face down and slides off the back. This really can happen, and besides being embarrassing, it hurts!

Many enclosed shopping malls open early to accommodate walkers. To find out about malls in your area, call the mall management office and ask if they open early for walkers. You should also ask if there are security officers on duty and what doors to the mall are open at that hour. Some malls actually provide

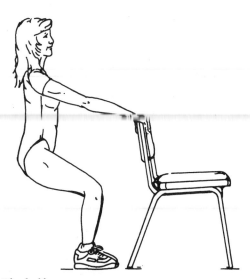

The half squat

maps to show the distances specific routes around the mall cover.

The next item on the agenda before you actually start walking is to get a good pair of shoes. You don't have to spend a lot of money, but it really makes a difference to your feet to have a good pair of walking shoes. Serious walking requires serious walking shoes, not casual canvas shoes with rubber soles and not shoes that were designed for other purposes like tennis or aerobics. Walking shoes and running shoes were specifically designed to give the feet the protection and support they need during the motion and impact of walking and running.

Now that you've picked a place and bought a good pair of shoes, you're ready to start your walking program. The ultimate goal of the walking program is to walk at a pace that is at least 3 mph (a 20-minute mile) for 50 minutes 5 times a week. Walking at 4 mph is even better and 5 mph is fantastic! However, I can't walk at a pace of 5 mph. For me, that's slow jogging. Jogging is not recommended for the woman with osteoporosis because of the impact loading of the spine. I want you to stay at a pace that will allow you to continue to walk. So there is some latitude here for the upper speed limit but the minimum speed is 3 mph. Your goal for endurance is 50 minutes.

Don't try to begin your exercise program with the final goals for speed and endurance. If necessary, start at a slower speed for a shorter period of time and gradually increase your speed and time over a period of weeks. For example, let's say you've decided to walk in your local mall. Pick a route around the mall of any distance you think you can walk without becoming overly tired, then walk that distance at a comfortable pace. Time yourself during the walk to see how long it takes you to do it. This first time out, you are not trying to walk any set distance at any set speed. You are just trying to see what you can reasonably and comfortably do. Once you have that information, you can begin to set some goals for yourself.

If you find that you can walk 50 minutes comfortably, then you will need only to concentrate on improving the speed at which you walk. On the other hand, if you walked at 3 mph or better but could only sustain that pace for a short period of time before needing to stop, your primary goal will be to improve your endurance. Most women need to work on both aspects, but one aspect may require more attention than the other. The speed program, the endurance program, and the combination speed-endurance program were designed by Phillip Walker, M.S.S., who is an exercise physiologist. Phillip is an exercise consultant at the Cooper Clinic with a special expertise in exercise in the prevention and treatment of osteoporosis.

THE SPEED PROGRAM

Let's say that you walked for 50 minutes and covered a distance of 1.7 miles, which is 0.034 miles per minute when divided by 50 minutes. Multiplying that figure by 60 tells you how many miles per hour you walked. This comes out to be 2 mph. If you walk at a pace of 3 mph, you should be able to cover that same 1.7 miles in only 34 minutes instead of 50 minutes. (Just remember the formula that speed multiplied by time equals distance.) Here's how a program to gradually increase your speed while continuing to walk for 50 minutes would work.

In your original walking session you walked 1.7 miles in 50 minutes for an average speed of 2 mph. For the first week of your walking program, you should continue to walk at your original pace, reaching the 1.7-mile mark in 50 minutes. Dur- ing week 2 on days 1, 3, and 5 of your 5-day exercise week, your goal will be to walk for 50 minutes as usual, but you must reach the 1.7-mile mark 2 minutes earlier than the week before. You should attempt to reach the 1.7-mile mark in 48 minutes instead of 50. Once you reach the 1.7-mile mark, continue to walk for 2 more minutes for a total of 50 minutes. On days 2 and 4 of your 5-day walking week, walk 50 minutes at whatever pace feels comfortable. Do not be concerned with your speed or distance.

On days 1, 3, and 5 of week 3 on this speed program your goal would be to reach the 1.7-mile mark in 46 minutes, instead of 48. Then continue to walk for 4 more minutes to reach your 50-minute total time goal. If you are unable to achieve the 1.7-mile mark in the allotted time of 46 minutes by the end of the third week, continue to strive for these same goals into the fourth week or as long as it takes to reach the 1.7-mile mark in 46 minutes. (Do not advance faster than 2 minutes per week.) Again, on days 2 and 4, walk at a comfortable pace for 50 minutes. In this example, if you were to progress by 2 minutes every week, it would take you 9 weeks to work up to a speed of 3 mph for 50 minutes. As you become comfortable with this pace, you will find that even on days 2 and 4, you will walk at the 3 mph pace without thinking about it. When you can walk for 50 minutes at a sustained pace of 3 mph, you will find that you are walking a total of 2.5 miles. In this same example, if you were to push to a pace of 4 mph, you would need to reach that same 1.7-mile mark in a time of 25.5 minutes. Increasing your pace in order to reach the 1.7-mile mark 2 minutes faster each week would result in reaching the 4-mph goal in 14 weeks. If you walk at a sustained pace of 4 mph, you would ulti-

mately cover 3.3 miles in 50 minutes. (4 mph × 50 min ÷ 60 min = 3.3 miles.)

To calculate how quickly you must reach your known distance to achieve the desired pace, do the following: Divide the known distance by the desired speed. Then multiply this number by 60. The result is the number of minutes you have to reach the distance you have measured to achieve the speed goal you have chosen. In the example I used above, to walk at a pace of 4 mph with the initial distance measured as 1.7 miles, the calculations were:

1. 1.7 miles divided by 4 mph equals 0.425 hours
2. 0.425 multiplied by 60 equals 25.5 minutes

If I reach the 1.7-mile mark in 25.5 minutes, I know that I have walked at a pace of 4 mph.

THE ENDURANCE PROGRAM

Let's say that during your initial trial walk you found that you walked 1 mile in 20 minutes. You had to stop at that point because you were too tired to continue. If you divide the distance you walked by the time, you will find that you were walking at a speed of 3 mph. (1 mile divided by 20 minutes equals 0.05 miles per minute multiplied by 60 minutes per hour equals 3 mph.) You just need to improve your endurance. Remember, your goal is to walk 50 minutes at a pace of at least 3 mph.

Like the speed program, I want you to try to improve by 2 minutes each week. During the first week, continue to walk 20 minutes at a pace of 3 mph as you did during the original session. On days 1, 3, and 5 of the second week, continue to walk at the pace of 3 mph but walk 22 minutes instead of 20. On days 2 and 4, walk at your 3-mph pace for whatever length of time is comfortable for you. During week 3 on days 1, 3, and 5, try to walk for 24 minutes—instead of 22 minutes—at the 3-mph pace. Again, on days 2 and 4, walk for whatever length of time is comfortable. Increasing your total walking time by 2 minutes each week means it will take 16 weeks to reach your goal of 50 minutes at 3 mph. I realize that this may seem like a long time. But this is the way to exercise safely. Your safety is of paramount importance, so don't be impatient.

THE COMBINATION SPEED AND ENDURANCE PROGRAM

Many women, particularly if they are recovering from an osteoporotic fracture, find that they can neither walk for a total of 50 minutes nor walk at a pace of 3 mph. Both speed and endurance must be improved. Both aspects of the walking program are approached gradually, just as they were in the speed program and in the endurance program.

On days 1 and 3 of your 5-day walking week, your goal is to increase your speed during your walk but not your total distance. You want to walk the same distance you did in your original session but walk that distance 1 minute faster than in the original session. Each week on days 1 and 3, you will be trying to walk the same original distance but 1 minute faster than the week before. Remember, the ultimate goal is to achieve a speed of at least 3 mph. Once you have reached a speed of 3 mph, you do not necessarily need to increase your speed further.

On days 2 and 4 of your 5-day exercise week, pay no particular attention to speed or distance. Simply walk a comfortable distance at a comfortable pace,

keeping in mind that your purpose in walking is exercise, not sight-seeing.

On day 5 of your exercise week, it is time to deliberately increase your total walking time. Walking at a comfortable pace, increase the amount of time you walk by 5 minutes each week. Your ultimate goal is a walk of 50 minutes. Once you have reached 50 minutes, you do not need to increase your walking time any more. During your second week of the program, the length of time you walk on day 5 will be 5 minutes longer than you walked in your original walking session. For subsequent weeks, this will be 5 minutes longer than you walked on day 5 of the previous week.

This walking program gradually builds endurance and strength by slowly increasing the speed and length of time you walk. Even though days 2 and 4 would be described as "free walking days," you will find that you walk faster and longer on these days as the program progresses because of your "speed" work on days 1 and 3 and your "endurance" work on day 5.

This isn't as complicated as it may sound. You will need to keep a record of your progress. A simple note pad will do, but you may opt to use a runner's diary, which can be purchased at most sporting goods or athletic shoe stores.

A SAMPLE COMBINATION ENDURANCE-SPEED WALKING PROGRAM

I developed this plan for one of my patients, Brenda S. Brenda is 65 years old and had experienced an osteoporotic spinal fracture 5 months before beginning this plan. Her pain had subsided sufficiently to allow her to begin a walking program.

Brenda's neighborhood was safe and convenient for her to use. There were paved sidewalks in every block and the terrain was relatively flat. On her first outing, Brenda found that she could walk 30 minutes before she became tired and experienced a recurrence of back pain. Her 30-minute walk allowed her to circle her block completely only one time. Although she now had her baseline values for the length of time to walk and the distance to walk, she could not be sure how fast she

BRENDA'S SECOND-WEEK WALKING VALUES

Day	Time	Distance	Emphasis
1	29 minutes	1 mile	Speed
2	Comfortable	Comfortable	None
3	29 minutes	1 mile	Speed
4	Comfortable	Comfortable	None
5	35 minutes	Not important	Endurance

BRENDA'S THIRD-WEEK WALKING VALUES

Day	Time	Distance	Emphasis
1	28 minutes	1 mile	Speed
2	Comfortable	Comfortable	
3	28 minutes	1 mile	Speed
4	Comfortable	Comfortable	
5	40 minutes	Not important	Endurance

BRENDA'S FOURTH-WEEK WALKING VALUES

Day	Time	Distance	Emphasis
1	27 minutes	1 mile	Speed
2	Comfortable	Comfortable	None
3	27 minutes	1 mile	Speed
4	Comfortable	Comfortable	None
5	45 minutes	Not important	Endurance

had walked without knowing the actual mileage for a trip around the block. To determine this, Brenda drove her car around the block, measuring the mileage with the car's odometer. (You can also use a trip meter, if your car has one.) She found that one trip around the block was 1 mile. She had walked 1 mile in 30 minutes, so she was able to calculate that she had walked at a speed of 2 mph. She could also calculate that if she walked at a pace of 3 mph, she should be able to walk 1 mile in only 20 minutes. Brenda now had all the information she needed to begin her walking program. During her first week of the walking program, Brenda continued to walk 30 minutes at a 2-mph pace on all 5 days. For the next few weeks, her program proceeded to improve.

As you can see, Brenda would reach her day-5 goal of a 50-minute walk by week 5. But it was going to take 11 weeks to reach the goal of walking 1 mile in 20 minutes on days 1 and 3.

Once Brenda reached the day-1 and day-3 goal of walking 1 mile in 20 minutes, which meant that she was walking at her goal pace of 3 mph, she then began the endurance program for days 1 and 3. In other words, on days 1 and 3 she would continue to walk at the 3-mph pace and increase the total time she walked by 2 minutes every week. It would take Brenda an additional 15 weeks to reach her goal of a 50-minute walk at 3 mph on days 1 and 3. She continued to walk on day 5 for 50 minutes at a comfortable pace. On days 2 and 4 she walked as long and as fast as she felt comfortable. She found that without really thinking about it, she was ultimately walking at a pace of 3 mph for 50 minutes 5 days a week at the end of week 26. It took Brenda 6 months to reach both her speed and endurance goals. However, she did reach it and she reached it *safely*.

PUMPING IRON

Of course you can do this, no, it's not unfeminine, and, yes, it is very beneficial. This is the last group of exercises to add to your osteoporosis exercise program. When should you add them? If you have had a fracture, I want you to wait until you are virtually pain free before beginning. Otherwise, when you find that you are capable of performing the chair extension exercises and the floor leg-lift, back-extension exercise twice a day for the maximum number of repetitions without pain, it's time to add some free weights or dumbbells to the program.

Free weights are dumbbells and barbells. These are the small, hand-held weights that you may have seen in gyms or fitness clubs. There are two basic types. A barbell is a small bar that weights of various sizes can be added to. A dumbbell is all one piece. The weights on this particular type of free weight are fixed. It is this latter type that I would prefer you use. The danger with the adjustable type of free weight is that the weight plates can slip off if not properly secured to the bar. (You will not need to constantly change the weights.) You will need a pair of free weights. They are often sold this way in sporting good stores. They come in shiny chrome, ugly black iron, and molded plastic in various designer colors. Shiny chrome is usually the most expensive and ugly black iron is the cheapest. Otherwise, the heavier the weight, the greater the cost. A 10-lb. weight will cost more than a 2-lb. weight. Most women are capable of using 3-lb. free weights, even when just beginning these exercises, and that is what I recommend. The best test, however, is to try lifting the weight in the store before you buy it. If you need a 2- or 1-lb. weight initially, that is fine.

These free-weight exercises emphasize strengthening of the arms, shoulders, and upper back. They are simple to perform, but it is important that you do the exercises properly. By and large, this means keeping the back straight during the performance of the exercise. Free-weight exercises are strength-training exercises, as we discussed in chapter 6. These exercises should be performed every other day, 3 days a week. Monday, Wednesday, and Friday or Tuesday, Thursday, and Saturday will do nicely.

The first free-weight exercise is called a bicep curl. Stand with the feet comfortably apart. Hold a weight in both hands. Your arms should be in front of your body with the palms facing forward. Rest your elbows against your body. Now raise your right arm, bending it at the elbow, and bring the weight up to your shoulder. Your elbow should remain against your body. Now lower the weight back down. Repeat with the left arm. You should raise the weight about twice as fast as you lower it. The muscle used in this exercise is the large muscle in the front of the upper arm, the bicep. Keeping your arms in front of your body with your elbow against your body is important. This ensures that you use only the bicep muscle to lift the weight and protects your elbow from being accidentally hyperextended when you lower the weight. As you perform the repetitions, remember to stand up straight with your chin up.

You need to continually check your posture while you perform these exercises—one reason that many people do these exercises in front of a mirror. The ultimate goal for the number of repetitions for the bicep curl is 25. Starting with 10 is appropriate.

Free-weight exercise number 2 is the wrist curl. You will need to sit down to perform this exercise. To exercise the right wrist, hold the weight in your right hand. Lay your forearm on your thigh with your palm up. Your forearm from elbow to wrist should be flat on your thigh. Allow your hand to fall down over your knee. In order to get your forearm flat, it is usually necessary to bend forward. That's okay, as long as you keep a little arch in your back while bending forward. Do not bend forward by rounding your back. Now, keeping your arm against your thigh, lift the

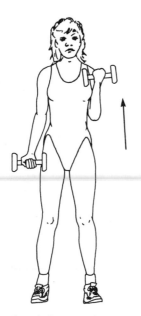

The bicep curl with free weights

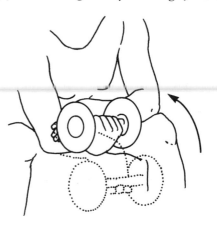

The wrist curl with free weights

weight by rolling your wrist up. Lower the weight back down. Repeat this wrist curl 25 times. As with the bicep curl, 10 repetitions is fine initially. Now repeat the exercise with the left wrist. The wrist curl exercises the muscles on the front of the forearm.

Now we need to exercise the muscles on the back of the forearm and upper arm. The opposite of the wrist curl is the wrist extension. This is usually more difficult than the wrist curl. If you are right handed, you will generally find that it is very difficult when exercising the left wrist. Don't get discouraged.

Just as for the wrist curl, for the wrist extension you are seated, bending forward with the back arched so that your forearm can lay flat on your thigh from wrist to elbow. To exercise your right wrist, again hold the weight in your right hand, but this time, roll your wrist over so that your palm is facing down allowing your hand to fall over your knee. Now lift the weight up, keeping your forearm on your thigh. Lower the weight back down. You may be able to repeat this exercise only 5 times initially. Your ultimate goal is 25, just as it is for the wrist curl and bicep curl. Repeat this exercise with the

left wrist. This is free-weight exercise number 3.

The triceps extension is free-weight exercise number 4. This is the exercise for the muscle on the back of the upper arm. Many women find this exercise more difficult than the bicep curl. The triceps extension exercise may be performed sitting or standing. Hold a free weight in one hand at a time. To perform a triceps extension with the right arm, hold the weight in your right hand. Now, lift your arm all the way up by the side of your head. Keeping your elbow up, allow your arm to bend at the elbow so that the weight is lowered to the back of your right shoulder. Keeping your elbow up and your arm close to your head, lift the weight up. Lift it gently. Don't jerk or pop the weight up. Your arm should be completely straight at the completion of the lifting motion. Now, carefully, lower the weight back down. Don't hit yourself in the back with the weight. Start with 5 or 10 repetitions for each arm with your goal being 25 repetitions for each arm. As you

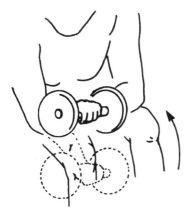

The wrist extension

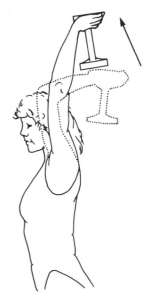

The triceps extension with free weights

perform the exercise, continually check your posture to be sure you are standing up straight. Again, a mirror comes in handy here.

If this seems too difficult or if you cannot control the weight enough to lower it gently, you can perform a two-handed triceps extension exercise. Hold the free weight with both hands much as you would hold a baseball bat. Raise both arms up, keeping them close to your head, and then lower the weight behind your head. Keep your elbows pointing up. Now, using both hands, raise the weight by straightening your arms. Again, be careful not to hit yourself in the back with the weight when you lower it.

The last free-weight exercise is number 5, the shoulder shrug. This exercise is just what it sounds like. Standing up tall, with your feet comfortably apart, hold a weight in each hand. Your arms should be at your sides and your palms facing your sides. Now, lift or shrug both shoulders at the same time. Lift them as high as they will go and then hold this position for a count of 3. Now lower your shoulders back down. The arms remain straight throughout the lift. As in every other exercise, lift the shoulders gently and smoothly. Don't jerk them up. This exercise will strengthen the muscles of the shoulders and upper back. Most women can perform at least 10 repetitions initially. The ultimate goal is, again, 25.

One pair of 3-lb. free weights will usually work well for all five exercises initially. Because the shoulder and upper back muscles are bigger than the arm muscles, even in those unaccustomed to lifting weights, you may find that you are ready for a heavier weight for the shoulder shrug fairly quickly. A 5-lb. weight could be used for this exercise once 25 repetitions can be performed with minimal effort. Similarly, once you can do 25 bicep curls with each arm without any difficulty, you can consider moving on to a 4- or 5-lb. free weight here. Many women have difficulty with a weight heavier than 3 lbs. in performing the remainder of the free-weight exercises.

These free-weight exercises are not intended to take the place of any of the back-extension exercises, stomach exercises, or any part of the walking program. They should be added to the program when you are ready to proceed. Like the back-extension exercises, they are not time consuming once you have learned how to do them. It's important that you realize that an exercise program is not just something else for you to do. It is as important to the success of your treatment as any prescription medication your doctor might give you for osteoporosis. Admittedly, it does require more effort and planning than taking a pill.

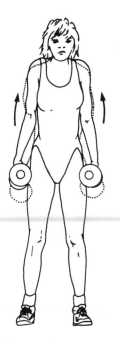

The shoulder shrug

PUTTING IT ALL TOGETHER

A woman who has had a fracture and still experiences pain should start with the chair extension exercises. Add the isometric abdominal exercises and leg-lift back-extension exercise as soon as the pain will permit. The walking program should be added next. A woman with osteoporosis who does not have any pain can begin both the walking program, back-extension exercises, and isometric abdominal exercises immediately. The free-weight exercises should be added to the exercise program last. Before adding these you should be pain free and capable of performing the maximum number of repetitions of the chair extension exercises and the floor leg-lift. If, on beginning the program, you can perform the maximum number of repetitions of these exercises, you may begin the free-weight program as well. If you experience any return of pain or increase in pain during the program, stop immediately and consult your physician.

CHAPTER 9

The Value of Vitamin D

Vitamin D is one of the most important vitamins the body needs for the bones. Vitamin D is often called the "sunshine vitamin" because the production of vitamin D by the body begins when the skin is exposed to sunlight. Ultraviolet radiation in sunlight reacts with a form of cholesterol in the skin called 7-dehydrocholesterol to produce a vitamin called pre-vitamin D. This pre-vitamin D undergoes some additional changes to become vitamin D_3. We can also get vitamin D_3 from foods and multivitamins. A slightly different vitamin D is vitamin D_2, which comes from plants. Vitamin D_2, which is found in food humans eat, is changed into vitamin D_3 in the body.

Vitamin D_3 doesn't really do much. In fact, there is some question as to whether it really does anything at all. In the liver, vitamin D_3 is changed into a form of vitamin D called 25 hydroxy-vitamin D_3. This is the most abundant form of vitamin D in the body. Twenty-five hydroxy-vitamin D_3 then goes to the kidney where it is changed again into 1,25 dihydroxy-vitamin D_3. As far as we know, it is this 1,25 dihydroxy-vitamin D_3 that is the active form of vitamin D. The vitamin D the kidney produces is the vitamin D that does the work.

Vitamin D (I am really referring to 1,25 dihydroxy-vitamin D_3, but for the sake of brevity I will call it vitamin D) has its most important effect on the intestinal tract. In the intestinal tract, vitamin D increases the absorption of calcium. For example, if the level of calcium in the blood dropped for some reason, a signal would be sent to the kidneys to produce more of the 1,25 dihydroxy-vitamin D_3 from the "liver" vitamin D, the 25 hydroxy-vitamin D_3. Increased amounts of the "kidney" vitamin D_3 are sent to the intestinal tract. More calcium is absorbed from the food and supplements and the level of calcium in the blood goes up. When the level of calcium in the blood goes up, the signal to the kidney to make "kidney" vitamin D_3 is turned off.

For this marvelous system to work, there must be an adequate supply of pre-vitamin D. The skin must be exposed to an adequate amount of sunshine and it must be able to make the pre-vitamin D from the cholesterol in the skin. Alternatively, an individual must consume an adequate amount of pre-vitamin D_3 or pre-vitamin D_2. The liver must be healthy enough to take the vitamin D_3 and turn it into the "liver" vitamin D and the kidney must be healthy enough to turn the "liver" vitamin D into the active "kidney" vitamin D. As you can see, all sorts of things could go wrong here. Fortunately, we can fix most of the problems that might occur.

Reasonably brief sunshine exposure is all that is necessary for the skin to make pre-vitamin D. Fifteen minutes a day is probably sufficient, resulting in the production of 100 to 200 units of vitamin D_3. Exposing the face, arms, and hands to early morning, midmorning, or late afternoon sun should provide ample stimulus to the skin without risking overexposure to the sun. A sunburn is absolutely unnecessary. You can't use a sunscreen during this time; it would prevent the skin from making vitamin D. The body can store this pre-vitamin D for that rainy day when you can't get any sunshine exposure.

Other circumstances may also prevent people from getting an average of 15 minutes of sunshine a day. In certain areas of the country in the wintertime, daylight hours are significantly shortened. Some authorities believe that in the northern part of the United States vitamin D deficiency in the winter may be much more common than we previously realized. Individuals who are hospitalized for long periods of time or who reside in nursing homes may receive no sun exposure at all. Research also indicates that as the skin ages, it loses some of its ability to make pre-vitamin D from sunshine exposure.

Only a few foods contain vitamin D_3 naturally. These are foods such as liver, fish, and egg yolks. In the United States some foods, such as milk, are fortified with vitamin D_3 or vitamin D_2. Vitamin D_3 is also found in multivitamins and combined with some calcium supplements. We certainly have access to vitamin D, but much as is the case with calcium, our vitamin D consumption declines dramatically with the elimination of milk from the diet. In addition, our ability to absorb vitamin D_3 from the diet appears to decline with age. Some diseases that affect the intestinal tract can result in an inability to absorb vitamin D from the diet.

If there is severe liver disease, the liver may be unable to take vitamin D_3 from the skin or diet and turn it into the "liver" vitamin D. Similarly, if there is severe kidney disease, the kidney may be unable to take the "liver" vitamin D and turn it into the active "kidney" vitamin D. After the age of 65, it also appears that the kidney's ability to make the "kidney" vitamin D tends to decline. Finally, there are some medications that increase the speed that the body eliminates vitamin D, making it less available for use by the body. Some of the medications we use to control seizures can do this.

The evidence that these factors are important in causing osteoporosis is strong. Measured levels of the "liver" vitamin D have been found to fall by more than 50% as we age. We know that after the age of 65, the measurable levels of the "kidney" vitamin D decrease by some 40%. The result is that the amount of calcium we absorb from the diet decreases by 40% between the ages of 20 and 80. In the wintertime, when sunshine exposure is limited and blood levels of vitamin D fall, bone loss has been shown to increase. Researchers in England found that patients with hip fractures had lower levels of the "liver" vitamin D than patients without hip fractures. On the other hand, research has now shown that supplementation with vitamin D combined with calcium reduces the risk of hip fracture in older individuals.

In December, 1992, in the *New England Journal of Medicine,* French researchers reported the results of a year-and-a-half long study of women who were given calcium and 800 units of vitamin D_3 compared with a group of women who received no calcium or vitamin D. At the end of the study, women taking 1,200 mg of calcium and 800 units of vitamin D_3 had 43% fewer hip fractures than the other women. In 1991, doctors from Tufts University reported that 400 units of vitamin D_3 combined with 377 mg of calcium resulted in a slowing of bone loss from the spine during the winter months when sunshine exposure was reduced.

. . . . research has now shown that supplementation with vitamin D reduces the risk of hip fracture in older individuals.

THE RDA FOR VITAMIN D

How much vitamin D do we need to adequately absorb the calcium from our diets? The RDA or recommended dietary allowance for vitamin D_3, like the RDA for calcium, depends on your age. Unlike calcium, however, we recommend the same amount for women as for men. Menopause has no effect on the RDA for vitamin D. The RDA for adults is 200 units.

The United States RDA for vitamin D is different. The U.S. RDA for adults is 400 units, not 200. **This greater amount of 400 units seems much more appropriate in light of the recent information on vitamin D.** In fact, some authorities recommend 800 units of vitamin D_3 for individuals over the age of 65.

It really isn't all that difficult to get adequate vitamin D. But if you routinely use a sunscreen on exposed skin, you cannot assume that you will produce vitamin D from sun exposure. In this case, or if you cannot be in the sun for 15 minutes a day, you must rely on dietary sources of vitamin D.

Much as is the case with calcium, concentrated sources of vitamin D in the diet are limited. If your sunshine exposure is too brief and your dietary sources of vitamin D are limited, a vitamin supplement is a reasonable alternative. Most multivitamins contain 400 units of vitamin D.

RECOMMENDED DAILY ALLOWANCE FOR VITAMIN D FROM THE NATIONAL ACADEMY OF SCIENCE	
Age	**International Units**
Children	
1–10	400
Adolescents and young adults	
11–24	400
Adults	
25+	200
During pregnancy	400
While breast feeding	400

Because the skin's ability to make vitamin D from sunshine exposure tends to decline with age and because the absorption of vitamin D from the intestinal tract also declines with age, I recommend a multivitamin containing 400 units of vitamin D to my patients over the age of 60.

DIETARY SOURCES OF VITAMIN D_3	
Food	**Units of Vitamin D**
Cod liver oil, 3.5 ounces	8,500
Margarine, 3.5 ounces	320
Raw herring, 3.5 ounces	900
Salmon, 3.5 ounces	600
Sardines in oil, 3.5 ounces	300
Chicken liver, 3.5 ounces	67
Milk, 1 cup	100
Egg, 1 whole	27
Swiss cheese, 3.5 ounces	100

> *. . . I recommend a multivitamin containing 400 units of vitamin D to my patients over the age of 60.*

I am often asked if you must take vitamin D with your calcium supplement. Many calcium supplements are combined with vitamin D. I have even heard people say that if vitamin D is not combined with the calcium supplement, you won't absorb the calcium. The answer to these questions lies in the knowledge that the vitamin D found in vitamins and combined with calcium supplements is vitamin D_3, which is inactive. (Remember, vitamin D_3 must be changed in the liver and then in the kidney before it becomes active in the body and helps you to absorb calcium.) So, while the vitamin D found in a vitamin or combined with a calcium supplement may help you absorb calcium tomorrow, it doesn't help you absorb the calcium you took today. That means that it is not necessary to take vitamin D at the same time as you take a calcium supplement. It also means that you do not have to take a combination calcium-vitamin D supplement to absorb the calcium.

> *. . . . you do not have to take a combination calcium-vitamin D supplement to absorb the calcium.*

The vitamin D found in multivitamins and in combination calcium supplements is the inactive vitamin D_3. You do not need a prescription to purchase these products because the amount of this inactive vitamin D is relatively small. There are occasions when a prescription form of vitamin D is required. Doctors have the ability to measure the level of vitamin D in the blood. We can measure the amount of "liver" vitamin D as well as the amount of "kidney" vitamin D. If an individual is found to be deficient in either of these types of vitamin D after a blood test, they can be given prescription versions of these types of vitamin D. Very large amounts of the inactive vitamin D_3 also require a prescription. The terminology here is quite confusing because the chemical names for all the different types of vitamin D are so similar. Cholecalciferol is the chemical name for inactive Vitamin D_3 made in the skin. Ergocalciferol is the chemical name for inactive vitamin D_2, which comes from plants. You can buy relatively high doses of inactive D_2 without a prescription. These should not be used unless you have been advised to do so by your physician. The liver-made vitamin D, or 25 hydroxy-vitamin D_3, is called calcefediol. It is sold only by prescription. The name of the prescription medication is called Calderol. The kidney-made vitamin D is called calcitriol. It is sold by prescription only under the name of Rocaltrol.

Excessive vitamin D can be dangerous. Vitamin D is stored in the body. Excessive amounts are not rapidly eliminated. Too much vitamin D can cause marked increases in the level of calcium in the blood, which can cause seizures, nausea, vomiting, and even death. That is why the more potent forms of vitamin D can only be bought with a prescription. Inactive vitamin D_2 or vitamin D_3 should not be taken in amounts greater than 1,000 units a day, except on the advice of a physician.

So get a little sunshine. Drink a glass of low-fat milk. A good multivitamin is a reasonable safeguard. If you are over 60, a multivitamin containing 400 units of vitamin D is essential.

Chapter 10

Examining Other Vitamins and Minerals

The science of nutrition is relatively new. We clearly do not know everything that we need to know. While medical authorities believe that vitamin D and the mineral calcium are critical to the development of strong, healthy bones, there may be other vitamins and minerals that are important as well. Research in this area is proceeding. It is worth looking at some of these new issues to see what is known and what is only speculation so that you can decide what is *both reasonable and safe* to do now to prevent osteoporosis.

Vitamins are organic molecules. They are generally needed in very small amounts. Vitamins can have multiple functions in the body. Many serve as catalysts or enzymes for the most basic and critical biochemical reactions in the body. If you pick up any bottle of multivitamins, you will find at least 12 or 13 vitamins listed in addition to vitamin D. Those vitamins that are thought to play a potential role in bone health are vitamins B_{12}, C, K, and A.

VITAMIN B_{12}

RDA for girls and women ages 11 and up: 2.0 micrograms.

Dietary sources: Muscle meats, eggs, dairy products. For example, 1 whole fresh egg contains 0.77 micrograms of B_{12}.

Some research suggests that vitamin B_{12} may be important for the osteoblasts, the cells that make new bone. Blood tests of alkaline phosphatase and osteocalcin, two substances found in bone that reflect new bone formation, are low in individuals with B_{12} deficiency. When treated with B_{12}, the levels promptly rise.

Unless your diet contains no muscle meat, eggs, or dairy products, it is next to impossible that you have a dietary deficiency of B_{12}. Certainly, an extreme vegetarian diet could produce B_{12} deficiency because B_{12} is not found in plant foods. B_{12} deficiency is a major feature of the disease pernicious anemia. B_{12} deficiency also occurs in persons who have undergone gastrointestinal surgery with complete or partial removal of the stomach or bypass of the stomach and small intestine. An enormous amount of vitamin B_{12} is stored in the liver, so it actually takes years of B_{12} deficiency before symptoms begin. No known disease results from excessive vitamin B_{12} ingestion.

At the present time, there does not seem to be any compelling reason to recommend vitamin B_{12} supplements as a general preventive measure in osteoporosis although B_{12} supplements are considered safe. Individuals who adhere to a strict vegetarian diet should consume a supplement to prevent the development of B_{12} deficiency. Those persons who have pernicious anemia or who have undergone gastrointestinal surgery, as noted above, will require injections of B_{12}.

VITAMIN K

RDA for girls 11–14: 45 micrograms
RDA for girls 15–18: 55 micrograms
RDA for women 19–24: 60 micrograms
RDA for women 25 and over: 65 micrograms

Dietary sources: green, leafy vegetables. There are small amounts in meats, cereals, and fruits. For example, 1 cup of lettuce contains 95 micrograms of vitamin K.

The evidence to support a role for vitamin K in bone health is based on the finding that vitamin K is required for the production of a bone protein called osteocalcin. Physicians can measure osteocalcin in the blood. Increased blood levels of osteocalcin are thought to mean that the bone cells are active, making new bone. The osteocalcin that is measured in the blood is osteocalcin that has "spilled over" from the bone. The exact function of osteocalcin within the bone itself is not known for sure. Researchers speculate that osteocalcin may in some way signal the bone to begin removing old bone, a process called resorption.

The most important, known role for vitamin K in the body is in the production of factors in the blood that are responsible for clotting. Individuals who are deficient in vitamin K may have bleeding problems. Given the limited information above, it seems quite premature to recommend that vitamin K be taken as a supplement to prevent osteoporosis. While vitamin K is relatively safe, excessive amounts of man-made forms of vitamin K can cause jaundice, a yellowing of the skin.

VITAMIN C

RDA for girls 11–14: 50 mg
RDA for girls and women 15 and over: 60 mg

Dietary sources: citrus fruits, green peppers, tomatoes, salad greens. For example, 1 medium orange contains about 60 mg of vitamin C.

Most people are familiar with scurvy, a disease that results from vitamin-C deficiency. Fortunately, scurvy is rare in Western societies. (It is still seen in infants who are fed a diet of boiled or pasteurized milk.) Osteoporosis can be caused by vitamin C deficiency and is seen in both infants and adults who have scurvy. Vitamin C is important in the production of a material called collagen. Collagen is perhaps best described as the fibrous tissue into which mineral is deposited in bone. Together with the mineral, collagen gives bone its strength. While it is clear that vitamin C is necessary for bone health, vitamin C deficiency is rare. Vitamin C supplementation as a general preventive measure for osteoporosis does not appear to be warranted. Vitamin C is also one of the vitamins that is often taken in megadoses in the United States because of the belief that it will prevent colds or other diseases. Excessive vitamin C is reported to cause certain types of kidney stones. In general, while meeting the RDA for vitamin C is beneficial and safe, excessive amounts of vitamin C are not recommended.

VITAMIN A

RDA for girls and women ages 11 and over: 800 micrograms in retinol equivalents or 8,000 units. (Vitamin A is really a group of substances that are chemically known as carotenoids, retinoids, retinol, retinaldehyde, and retinoic acid. The activity of these substances in the body is not the same. In order to compare the strength of one substance with another, a standard of vitamin A activity, called a retinol equivalent, is used.)

Dietary sources: green vegetables, milk, butter, and cheese. For example, $^2/_3$ cup of cooked broccoli contains 2,500 units of vitamin A.

Vitamin A is also popularly known today as beta-carotene. Beta-carotene is actually a precursor to vitamin A. Vitamin A is considered critical to normal growth of the skeleton, but excessive vitamin A poses real dangers. Vitamin A intoxication causes weakness, fatigue, emotional disturbances, headache, and aching in muscles and bone. Unfortunately, vitamin A is also one of the vitamins often taken in excess in the United States because of recent reports suggesting its beta-carotene content may protect against cancer. As far as osteoporosis prevention is concerned, vitamin A supplementation is not recommended. In general, while meeting the RDA for vitamin A is reasonable, consuming amounts in excess of the RDA is not recommended.

OTHER MINERALS AND TRACE ELEMENTS

The most important minerals in nutrition are calcium, phosphorus, magnesium, iron, zinc, and iodine. Trace elements include copper, fluoride, chromium, selenium, molybdenum, manganese, boron, and aluminum. Deficiencies in some of these minerals and elements, other than calcium, have been linked to osteoporosis, notably magnesium, zinc, boron, and manganese. Excess fluoride has been implicated in the cause of osteoporosis as well as being lauded as a treatment. Let's briefly look at the evidence to determine what is both reasonable and safe under the circumstances.

MAGNESIUM

RDA for girls 11–14: 280 mg
RDA for girls 15–18: 300 mg
RDA for women 19 and over: 280 mg

Dietary sources: Whole grains; green, leafy vegetables. For example, 1 cup of cooked spaghetti has 29 mg of magnesium.

The average adult has about 25 g of magnesium in the body and half of that is found in the bones. That fact alone would make one wonder if we should pay more attention to the amount of magnesium we consume to prevent osteoporosis. Medical science used to say that magnesium deficiency was rare and only occurred in individuals who were truly malnourished or had specific diseases like alcoholism. We now know that some diuretics can cause an excess loss of magnesium. These diuretics are in the family of medications called thiazides. Thiazide diuretics are often prescribed for high blood pressure, heart failure, and fluid retention. Part of the problem in identifying true magnesium deficiency lies in the fact that, although we can measure magnesium in the blood, the blood level does not accurately reflect the depletion of magnesium stored in the body until that depletion is quite profound. So even if the blood magnesium level is normal, many physicians are now adding a magnesium supplement to the treatment of patients who must take these kinds of diuretics.

But do you need a magnesium supplement as a general preventive measure in osteoporosis? Most of the research that has been used to support the use of magnesium supplements in osteoporosis prevention has relied on the finding that osteoporosis is more common in patients who have other diseases known to cause magnesium deficiency like alcoholism, diabetes, and hyperthyroidism. But this doesn't prove cause and effect. It only suggests an association. In fact, when the magnesium content of bones from patients with osteoporosis has been analyzed, more magnesium than usual has been found in those bones.

Magnesium does play a role in the control of the production of a bone hormone called parathyroid hormone. If magnesium is deficient, less parathyroid hormone is released. The net result of this would seem to be less bone loss, not more. There is a great deal of research on magnesium at present but no single opinion as to what all this research means.

Individuals who have diseases or who must take medications that can cause magnesium loss should take a magnesium supplement if directed to do so by their physicians. Recommending magnesium supplements for the general prevention of osteoporosis in otherwise healthy individuals does not appear to be appropriate. Too much magnesium can be unpleasant. Excessive magnesium will cause diarrhea. You have probably experienced this if you have ever taken a laxative such as Milk of Magnesia.

ZINC

RDA for girls and women 11 and over: 12 mg.

Dietary sources: small amounts in all types of foods.

Zinc is an essential element in human nutrition and there is no question that zinc deficiency causes disease. Stunted growth and defective production of proteins result from zinc deficiency. Even though zinc is found in small amounts in many different types of foods, it is widely believed to be inadequate or, at best, marginal in most Western diets. What is the evidence that zinc deficiency may play a role in the development of osteoporosis?

A significant amount of the zinc in the body is found in bone. In conditions that are known to result in bone loss, increased amounts of zinc are found in the urine. Some researchers have used the amount of zinc in the urine as a test to detect rapid bone loss. The increased zinc in the urine is a result of the bone loss. Can zinc deficiency cause bone loss in the first place? That is obviously a different question. As noted above, zinc deficiency does result in stunted growth in children. Low blood levels of zinc have been found in patients with osteoporosis. Zinc may directly affect the bones' ability to make new bone or it may affect how the bone responds to other hormones that control bone loss and bone gain. The information on zinc, while not indicating a need to consume more zinc than the amount listed as the RDA, is compelling enough to strongly suggest careful attention to meeting the RDA for zinc. The best advice, of course, is to eat a well-balanced diet. Perhaps more realistic advice is to use a good multivitamin plus mineral preparation that contains 12 mg of zinc.

MANGANESE

RDA is not established. Instead, a desirable intake range, which is 2.5–6.0 mg for children and adults ages 11 and over is used.

Dietary sources: widely distributed in different food types.

Manganese is considered a trace element. We need very small amounts of this element for proper nutrition, which is why it is called a "trace" element. Another property of trace elements is that toxic levels of trace elements may be only two or three times the recommended intake level, so caution is clearly advised before adding trace element supplements in amounts that exceed the recommended intake range.

Manganese deficiencies can cause disease. Manganese does appear to be critical to the proper development of cartilage and bone. Although much of the research has been in chickens and rats, not human beings, osteoporosis has been reported in people who were deficient in manganese. These individuals were also deficient in several other minerals and elements as well, so we cannot be entirely sure of the significance of the manganese deficiency. Perhaps the most celebrated case of manganese deficiency was in a well-known professional athlete (Bill Walton) who suffered repeated fractures that would not heal while playing basketball. This young man was also deficient in other minerals. These deficiencies were attributed to the bizarre, highly restricted diet he had been consuming.

Manganese has actually replaced lead in gasoline. The relevance of this to the diet is that there are now increased amounts of manganese in the air as a pollutant of sorts. That should actually result in increased amounts of manganese in food, making dietary manganese deficiency unlikely. Excessive manganese can produce a generalized disease of the nervous system. All things considered, it would seem unwise and unnecessary to deliberately supplement a relatively normal diet with increased amounts of manganese for the prevention of osteoporosis.

BORON

RDA not established. Recommended range of intakes not established. Customary intake in American diets is 1 to 3 mg a day.

Dietary sources: fruits and vegetables.

You can see that we really don't know how much, if any, boron we should be consuming. And yet, boron is being recommended as both a preventative and cure for osteoporosis in some health-food stores. This recommendation is based predominantly on one study in postmenopausal women in which boron supplementation of 3 mg a day was given while the women were on a boron-deficient diet. Estrogen and testosterone levels in these women increased and the amount of calcium lost in the urine decreased.

Other research studies have not been able to confirm these findings. The bulk of research on boron's effect on bone has been done in rats, rabbits, chickens, and cattle. It would seem premature to conclude that boron is either a cure or a means of preventing osteoporosis in people and so I do not recommend the use of specific boron supplements. Most multivitamin and mineral combination supplements do not contain boron or contain very small amounts that are safe. For example, Centrum, a multivitamin and mineral preparation made by Lederle, contains only 150 micrograms of boron. Excessive boron is toxic.

COPPER

RDA not established. Recommended range of intake for children and adults age 11 and over is 2 to 3 mg a day.

Dietary sources: meats, particularly white meats, and water.

There are diseases in which copper deficiency is clearly associated with osteoporosis. Some of these diseases are due to the inherited inability to absorb copper from the diet. Dietary copper deficiency has not been directly linked to postmenopausal osteoporosis, although it has been linked to abnormalities in the bones of children and infants.

Indirect evidence for a role of copper deficiency in postmenopausal osteoporosis comes from one research study that suggested that women with hip fractures from osteoporosis had lower copper levels than women without hip fractures of the same age. This does not prove that copper deficiency caused the fractures. We do not know if copper deficiency really causes or contributes to postmenopausal osteoporosis. Researchers speculate that copper deficiency might decrease our defense against what are called free radicals. Free radicals have been identified as causing bone loss. This must still be con-

sidered only theory at this point in time. Just to confound the experts, copper excess is also associated with bone abnormalities. Specific copper supplements are not currently recommended to prevent osteoporosis. Most multivitamin plus mineral preparations will contain 2 mg of copper.

SILICON

RDA is not established.

Dietary sources: widely distributed in foods.

Silicon is another trace element. Although silicon is touted in some health-food stores as a means of preventing osteoporosis, no documented cases of osteoporosis have been caused by silicon deficiency or cured by silicon treatment. Silicon is essential in animals for proper bone development. In laboratory studies, silicon seems to have an effect on bone formation. Good scientific information on silicon is still quite limited; it is extremely premature to recommend silicon supplementation.

FLUORIDE

RDA is not established. Recommended range of intake is 1.5–2.5 mg for children ages 11 and over and 1.5–4.0 mg a day for adults.

Dietary sources: water, seafood, tea.

In the 1940s it was noted that mine workers repeatedly exposed to fluoride dust developed a painful bone disease called fluorosis, in which the bones became very dense. In studying this disease, it was found that fluoride could actually increase the number of osteoblasts, the bone-forming cells, which resulted in the formation of more bone. It was also found that fluoride could become part of the crystal structure of bone itself. While the bone in individuals who developed fluorosis was clearly abnormal bone, researchers speculated that carefully controlled amounts of fluoride might be beneficial to the bone and perhaps even useful in treating osteoporosis.

Fluoride is added to drinking water in many communities to prevent dental cavities. Fluoride tablets can also be prescribed by dentists for the same purpose. But fluoride's role in either the prevention or treatment of osteoporosis remains both controversial and investigational. Excessive fluoride is clearly harmful, producing mottling of the teeth, abnormal bone, and neurologic problems. In research studies that have used fluoride to treat osteoporosis, dramatic increases in spinal bone density occurred but fractures continued to occur, suggesting that the quality of the new bone was poor. Researchers have also noted an increase in hip fractures in patients treated with fluoride, although this has not been conclusively proven to be the result of fluoride treatment. Medical science is still trying to find a way to safely harness fluoride's ability to increase the bone density in the spine. Fluoride is a very intriguing mineral. At present, its use in the prevention and treatment of osteoporosis should be confined to carefully controlled research studies. Fluoride supplementation to prevent osteoporosis is not recommended at this time.

SHOULD YOU EVER TAKE EXTRA VITAMINS AND MINERALS?

I do. I take a multivitamin plus mineral supplement every day. I use a major brand that is available without a prescription. It provides me with 100% of the RDA for all the major vitamins and minerals. Why? Because I know that most nutritionists would cringe at my usual diet. I am not good about getting enough servings of fresh fruits and vegetables and I often eat on the run. Hopefully, your diet is better than mine. I know that there is no harm in a multivitamin plus mineral supplement that supplies 100% of the RDAs so this is safe for me to do. Most women will also need a calcium supplement because of calcium-deficient diets due to the limited sources of calcium in the diet. Manufacturers cannot generally put enough calcium into a vitamin plus mineral supplement to meet this need because the tablet would be too big to swallow. Some women will also need an iron supplement because of the iron lost with each menstrual period. I recommend a vitamin D supplement (a good multivitamin is fine) for my patients over 65. It's also reasonable to recommend a multivitamin plus mineral supplement during periods of stress and illness because it may help the body cope with these periods. I do not recommend you take amounts of vitamins and minerals that greatly exceed the RDAs or recommended intake ranges unless your doctor prescribes this as part of the treatment of a specific disease. The benefits of doing so are only speculative at best and there can be real potential harm.

CHAPTER 11

Preventing Falls

Often, when I sit down to talk with my patients about preventing falls at home, they begin to look despondent. They seem to think that this is a last-ditch effort to prevent them from breaking a bone because there is nothing else that can be done for them. Nothing could be farther from the truth! I simply am a firm believer in the old adage "an ounce of prevention is worth a pound of cure."

In an average year, 20% to 30% of people over the age of 65 will fall. Of people over the age of 80, some 50% will fall at least once. Many osteoporotic fractures are the result of falls. Wrist fractures, pelvic fractures, and, tragically, hip fractures are often the result of falls that could have been prevented. In contrast, spinal fractures occur during ordinary activities that require bending, stooping, or lifting. Five to 10% of falls result in serious injuries other than fractures. In fact, accidental deaths, most of which are due to falls, are the sixth leading cause of death in the elderly. According to the National Safety Council, 74% of all deaths due to falls in 1987 were in people 65 years of age or older. The National Osteoporosis Foundation in Washington, DC, states that 50,000 deaths occur each year from hip fractures that result from falls. Falling is also listed as a contributing factor in 40% of nursing home admissions.

Why do we fall? In the late nineteenth century, a German physician noted that women fell and broke their hips more often than men. He thought it was because

women were tripping over the hems of their long skirts. Thank goodness hems have risen over the years. But we are still falling, and women fall more often than men. Why?

> *In an average year, 20% to 30% of people 65 years of age and older will fall.*

In a recent study published in the *Annals of Internal Medicine*, people who had recently fallen were studied to determine why they fell. Some of the major causes were muscle weakness and poor coordination, environmental hazards, dizziness or light-headedness when standing, and medication-related side effects. All of these factors can and should be addressed. The place to start is where most falls occur—the home.

HOME SWEET HOME

Preventing falls, particularly in the home, requires more common sense than anything else. It is worth discussing some points that may be so simple that we don't think of them.

The most dangerous room in the house is the bathroom. Almost everyone, regardless of age, has slipped in the bath or shower at least once. If you were lucky, you caught yourself before you fell. It's not

119

a sign of old age or infirmity to reduce the risk of falling in the bathroom. It's just good sense!

The most important change you can make in your bathroom is to install safety, or "grab," bars in the tub and shower. Safety bars have been used in hospitals for years. And for years, they looked like they belonged in hospitals. They were large, stainless steel bars which no one would particularly want gracing the bath in his or her house. Now safety bars that match or complement your decor are available. The bars come in different lengths and can be installed vertically, horizontally, or at an angle to meet your specific needs.

So where do you need them? Again, a little common sense seems in order. Generally speaking, falls occur when a person is either stepping in or out of the tub. Falls also occur as a person sits down or stands up in the tub. It will likely take three bars, properly placed, to protect you from these types of falls in the bath.

The first bar should be placed vertically on the side wall of the tub enclosure to aid in stepping into the tub. The second bar should be placed vertically on the wall outside of the tub enclosure to aid in stepping out of the tub. Don't be tempted to think that the towel rack, which is often found in this same location, can substitute. It is not meant to hold your weight and would rip out of the wall if you were to grab it. The last bar should be placed on the back wall of the tub at an intermediate height so that it can be reached in the sitting position. This bar can be placed vertically as well or can be placed at a 45-degree angle. An L-shaped bar is also available and is quite useful in this location.

These bars are not terribly expensive. They range in price from $16 to $27. Safety bars are available in hardware stores and from medical equipment supply dealers. Several types of safety bars are

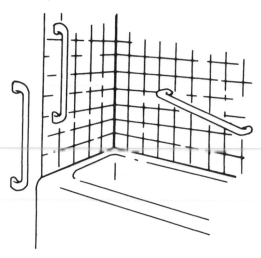

Correctly installed safety bars

available by mail order from North Coast Medical, Inc., a medical equipment supply dealer in San Jose, California. (See the appendices for the address and phone number.) Check with dealers in your area as well for price comparisons and quality of the merchandise.

Once you have purchased the bars, don't skimp on the installation. It is imperative that the bars be installed properly so they will provide the support you need if you fall. The bars generally come with long screws that must be inserted into the studs inside the wall. If the screws are not placed into the studs, the bar may pull out of the wall when you try to support your weight with the bar. A professional plumber or carpenter can install the bars if this seems too difficult. The cost of an hour of labor from a plumber or carpenter obviously increases the cost of this prevention measure. But remember, a hip fracture can cost a life.

A final touch to the bath is to install nonskid rubber mats or strips on the floor of the tub to improve traction. Once this is done, you will have made the bath as safe as you possibly can.

Having gone to this length to make the bathtub safe, don't undermine these

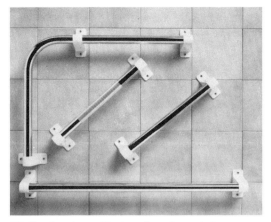

Wall safety bars. Various lengths and shapes allow for optimum placement in the tub or shower to reduce the risk of falling. Photo courtesy of North Coast Medical, Inc., San Jose, California.

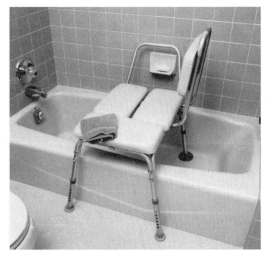

Tub transfer bench. The bench allows an individual to sit down and then slide over into the tub. This is useful for someone who is too weak to step into the bath or to sit down in the tub. Photo courtesy of North Coast Medical, Inc., San Jose, California.

precautions by putting bath oils in the water. Bath oils and water softeners make the surface of the tub very slippery and increase the likelihood of falls. If you wish, use a bath oil or lotion that is applied after the bath.

A final accessory that may be useful is a bath chair or bath bench. This is for the individual who either has great difficulty in sitting down or standing up in the tub or for the individual who cannot stand for an adequate length of time during a shower. Bath benches, like safety bars, can be purchased from hardware stores and medical equipment supply stores. Prices range from $30 to $80. More expensive, but often very useful for the older individual, is a transfer bench. These benches actually extend out over the side of the tub. The individual sits down outside the tub and then slides over onto the tub portion of the bench. North Coast Medical, Inc., sells one of the available transfer benches for around $130.

Shower enclosures that are separate from the tub should also be inspected to assess the danger of falling. If possible, safety bars should be placed both inside and outside of the enclosure to aid in entering and exiting. If it is not possible to place a bar inside the enclosure, nonskid rubber strips on the floor should certainly be used to improve traction.

Falls also occur in the home in the middle of the night, when an individual gets up to go to the bathroom or kitchen. Two contributing elements need to be addressed: the darkness and the path.

Most of us simply get up in the dark and make our way by memory, still half asleep, to the bath or kitchen. We rarely turn on a light because we don't want to wake other family members or because we want to avoid that sudden shock of bright light. Night-lights, installed in just a few locations, can sufficiently brighten these areas without disturbing sleep and make this short journey much safer. I prefer the type of night-light that stays on all the time (or one that has a light sensor and turns on automatically) rather than one you must turn on manually, unless you intend to leave it on all the time. While that may sound wasteful, night-lights use very little energy and are absolutely useless if you forget to turn them on before you go to bed.

Items that might cause you to trip should not be left on the floor. Children's toys, clothing, boxes, etc., should all be moved out of the traffic pattern to the bath and kitchen, even if they are not really put away until the following day.

The next most dangerous room in the house is the kitchen. Again, this is an area of the home where floor surfaces may become slippery. You should make it a habit to wipe up any spills immediately. (And certainly, as both a woman and a physician, it seems to me that the prevention of falls is an excellent reason not to mop or wax the kitchen floor.) Do what you must in this regard, but be careful.

One more simple and often overlooked preventive measure in the kitchen is to rearrange the storage space. Items and appliances that are frequently used should be stored on counters or shelves that are easily reached without the aid of a stepladder or stool.

Area rugs are another major cause of falls in the home. Area rugs, particularly small ones, can slip. Toes are often caught on the edge of the rug. Both can, and often do, result in falls. My own preference is to remove area rugs from the home. If you choose to keep them, use the available nonskid mats and backing materials to prevent slipping. The edges of the rug still pose a hazard.

Finally, if there are any stairs or steps leading into or within the house, handrails should be installed at each location. Cracks in sidewalks should be patched and entryways should be well lit at night.

Making these modifications within the home is not meant to make you paranoid about falling. Most of these changes

are things you do once. Then they are always there for you to use when you need them.

HOUSE SHOES

Complaints about women's shoes could fill another book. In the context of reducing the risk of falling, a word should be said about house shoes or slippers. There are two things to avoid: platform-style slippers and slippers with fabric soles. Any slipper or house shoe should have a back that comes up over the heel like a moccasin or loafer-style shoe. The platform-style slipper makes it very easy for your heel to slip off the back of the shoe, which can result in a fall, particularly in the older individual whose balance may be impaired.

The soles of house shoes should be nonskid rather than soft fabric. Fabric-sole shoes, particularly on vinyl surfaces like those found in the kitchen or bath, slip very easily.

If you have already taken most of these steps to protect yourself, have you considered what your parents or grandparents might need? A new pair of slippers is an inexpensive gift. Although installing safety bars in the bathroom might seem like a strange birthday or anniversary present, it just might be the best gift you ever gave them.

EYESIGHT AND DIZZINESS

Besides the environment in which we live, there are other common causes of falling that can be addressed if they are recognized. In older individuals, failing eyesight can contribute to the risk of falling. Nearsightedness, far-sightedness, or cataracts should not go untreated. A check-up with an ophthalmologist or optometrist to see if a prescription for glasses or other treatment is needed may be in order.

Postural dizziness, which is dizziness upon standing, is common in people over 65. In one study of almost 10,000 women over 65, 19% of the women complained of postural dizziness. In this same study, postural dizziness was also found to be a risk factor for falling. If you or a member of your family has complained of this, see your doctor for an evaluation. In the meantime, stand up slowly. Once up, stand still for just a few seconds before you start to walk.

MEDICATIONS

Some types of medication can increase the risk of falls. These medications are often prescribed for very valid reasons, but can cause drowsiness, dizziness, and poor coordination. The most commonly used

drugs that may have these side effects are long-acting sleeping pills and tranquilizers, some antidepressants, and drugs called antipsychotics, which are used to treat serious mental illnesses. Not surprisingly, the larger the dose of these types of medications, the greater the risk of falling.

I do not mean to imply that these drugs are bad or that they should not be used. They have important and necessary roles in treating illness. If your doctor has prescribed any of these medications for you, *do not stop taking them without talking with him or her first*. But it is important that you are aware that these types of medications can increase the risk of falling so that you can take the proper precautions.

MUSCLE WEAKNESS

Muscle weakness, poor coordination, and a lack of agility can all be improved or eliminated with exercise, regardless of age. Exercise programs are discussed at length in chapters 7 and 8.

AN OUNCE OF PREVENTION . . .

The prevention of falls, particularly for an older individual, is as important as any other osteoporosis-prevention measure. Although spinal fractures can occur during the performance of ordinary activities if the bones are weak, hip fractures and wrist fractures are usually caused by falls—falls that could have been prevented. Beyond the immediate pain and suffering caused by a hip fracture is the loss of physical independence and even loss of life that may result. The simple steps outlined in this chapter can help prevent this tragedy.

COMMONLY USED MEDICATIONS THAT CAN CAUSE DROWSINESS OR IMPAIR BALANCE AND COORDINATION

Trade Name	Generic Name
Dalmane	Flurozepam
Valium	Diazepam
Librium	Chlordiazepoxide
Elavil	Amitriptyline
Sinequan	Doxepin
Tofranil	Imipramine
Mellaril	Thioridazine
Haldol	Haloperidol
Thorazine	Chlorpromazine

CHAPTER 12

Bone-Density Testing

The term "bone density" means the amount of mineral contained within a certain amount of bone. For example, you might have 1 g of mineral for every square centimeter of bone. So, your bone mineral density or BMD would be 1.0 g/cm^2. The bone mineral density is important because it is the density that largely determines how strong your bones are. Another way of looking at it is that your bone mineral density determines how likely you are to have an osteoporotic fracture.

The ability to actually measure the bone density is relatively new. We have been able to see the bones with regular medical X rays for quite some time, but that never really helped us determine how strong the bones were. It is true that the more dense (in this context, strong and dense mean the same thing) the bones are, the whiter they will appear on an X ray. But the whiteness or blackness of the images on an X ray is also determined by the exposure settings on the X-ray machine, much as the lightness and darkness of a photograph are determined by the settings on a camera. The very subtle changes in the whiteness of the bones that occur as bone is lost cannot be seen by the human eye on a regular X ray until a great deal of bone has been lost.

REGULAR X RAYS

When a doctor X rays your spine, for example, he or she will not notice any real difference in how white the bones are until you have lost at least 30% of your bone density. If bone loss is suspected from a regular X ray based on the whiteness of the bones (or lack of it), the best we can say is that at least 30% of the bone density, and possibly more, is already gone. It is not possible to detect small amounts of bone loss or to accurately assess bone strength with a regular X ray. There is no way to predict an individual's risk of having a fracture in the future from a regular X ray.

THE USE OF RISK FACTORS

Doctors have tried to predict which women might be at a greater risk of having an osteoporotic fracture in the future by asking them about risk factors for osteoporosis. Risk factors (see chapter 2) are useful. You definitely want to identify those risk factors you can change and get rid of them—correct calcium deficiency, reduce caffeine, exercise regularly, stop smoking, and so on. This will help to reduce your risk of osteoporosis. Unfortunately, there will always be some risk factors that you cannot eliminate. You cannot change the fact that you are Hispanic, Caucasian, or Asian. You cannot change the fact that your mother or grandmother had osteoporosis. And you cannot change the fact that you have entered menopause.

But can your doctor really predict, based on the presence or absence of these risk factors, what your bone density is now? Can he or she predict that you will develop an osteoporotic fracture based on your risk factors? Using a woman's answers to a series of questions about risk factors to decide if she is truly at risk for osteoporosis turns out to be no better than flipping a coin!

A group of doctors from Toulouse, France, published an interesting study in 1991 in which they asked 2,279 women who had been referred to a menopause clinic a series of questions designed to identify 18 different risk factors for osteoporosis. The doctors also measured the bone density in these women's spines. Fifty-four percent of the women whose bone density was low—putting them at high risk for osteoporotic fracture—had no risk factors for osteoporosis other than the fact that they were women. The doctors concluded that risk-factor questionnaires were not a reliable means of identifying women at risk for osteoporosis. So how can we identify women at risk? By measuring the bone density.

SINGLE PHOTON ABSORPTIOMETRY (SPA)

Bone-density measurements have actually been available for some time but early technologies were limited in their usefulness. The modern era of bone-density testing really began in the 1960s. A technique called single photon absorptiometry, or SPA, was introduced in clinical medicine. The nature of SPA was such that it could only measure the bone density in the bones of the skeleton that were not surrounded by large amounts of muscle or other tissue. That effectively limited SPA to measurements of the wrist and, years later, the heel.

Identification of the woman who is at risk for wrist fracture is important. But an SPA measurement of the wrist in the early years of use could not give us much insight into what was happening in the spine and hip where the more serious fractures occur. We needed a way to look directly at the spine and the hip so that we could learn how to protect those areas of

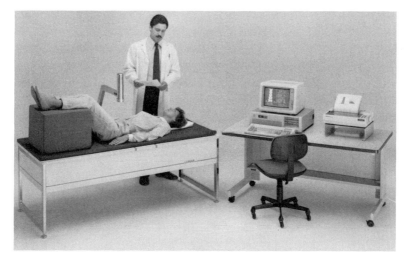

Dual Photon Absorptiometry or DPA. This is an early DPA machine. This woman is having a spine bone density measurement performed.
Photo courtesy of LUNAR, Madison, Wisconsin.

125

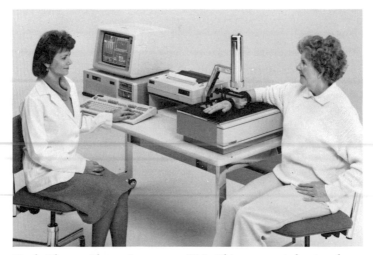

Single Photon Absorptiometry or SPA. This woman is having the density of her wrist bone measured. Photo courtesy of LUNAR, Madison, Wisconsin.

the skeleton and find the women who were at risk for spinal and hip fracture.

DUAL PHOTON ABSORPTIOMETRY (DPA)

In the late 1970s and early 1980s, significant advances were made with the introduction of dual photon absorptiometry, or DPA. With DPA, we could measure the bone density in the spine and hip. DPA ultimately advanced to the point that the entire body could be measured to give the doctor an assessment of total body bone mineral density.

Both SPA and DPA used radioactive materials inside the machines. Although that may sound dangerous, it was not. It did make the machine upkeep more expensive. The radioactive material in a single photon absorptiometer had to be replaced every 6 months. The radioactive material in a DPA machine had to be replaced about once a year at a cost of $5,000 to $7,000 every time.

There has never been any question about the safety of SPA or DPA tests. A patient having a test with either SPA or DPA is exposed to radiation, but the amount of exposure is extremely small. During a DPA spine test, the radiation is only $1/12$ of the radiation given during a front- and side-view chest X ray. The radiation to the wrist during an SPA study was about $1/4$ of the chest X ray, but no vital organs were exposed to the X ray during the study.

> *. . . . risk-factor questionnaires were not a reliable means of identifying women at risk for osteoporosis.*

DPA was a major advance because we could finally measure the bone density in the spine and hip. It does have two limitations. First, it is relatively slow. A study of the spine takes about 25 minutes. A study of the hip might take 35 or 40 minutes. If your doctor orders a total body bone-density study, that can take over an hour. Some patients don't find that an inconvenience. The test is not at all unpleasant and many patients simply take a short nap.

From the medical point of view, the main limitation of DPA involves the precision of the test. Don't misunderstand. DPA can accurately measure the bone density in the spine, hip, and total body. The risk of having a fracture can be predicted from that measurement. The limitation of DPA is in its ability to detect small changes in the bone density over time. This is called precision. The precision of DPA just isn't good enough so that your doctor can measure your bone density today and again in a year and know if you have lost 1%, 2%, 3%, or 4% of your bone in that period of time. If you have lost 10% or 15% of your bone density, that will be obvious, but we can't be sure about the smaller changes with only two measurements 1 year apart.

Dual Energy X-ray Absorptiometry (DEXA or DXA)

In 1988, the FDA approved the most significant advance in bone-density technology to date: dual energy X-ray absorptiometry, or DEXA (the abbreviation DXA is also used). With DEXA, there is no radioactive isotope in the machine. The machine uses an X-ray tube and is controlled by a computer. With DEXA, virtually every area of the skeleton can be measured: the spine, hip, wrist, heel, arms, legs, and the entire body. DEXA combines, and surpasses the abilities of SPA and DPA. DEXA is incredibly fast. Instead of a 20-minute spine study, as was done with DPA, DEXA machines can do the same

test in 2 to 4 minutes. A hip study with DEXA also takes only 2 to 4 minutes instead of 35 or 40. A total-body study can be done in only 10 minutes. There are also new machines on the way that are even faster.

> *In 1988, the FDA approved the most significant advance in bone-density technology to date: dual energy X-ray absorptiometry, or DEXA.*

Accuracy has not been sacrificed in the interest of speed. The tests are highly accurate. Equally important, radiation exposure has been reduced. A spine study or hip study is now $1/30$ of the radiation of a front- and side-view chest X ray. I certainly don't mean to minimize the issue of radiation exposure during a test. Any radiation exposure should be carefully considered in advance. But to put this in proper perspective, the radiation exposure during

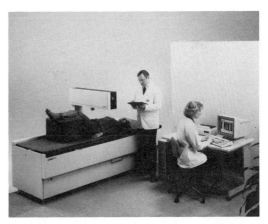

Dual Energy X ray Absorptiometry or DEXA. DEXA is now considered the technique of choice (to measure bone density) by many authorities. Photo courtesy of LUNAR, Madison, Wisconsin.

a DEXA spine study is the same or less than the radiation exposure to a passenger on a trans-Atlantic airline flight. Certainly going to Europe is more enjoyable than a DEXA study, but neither is dangerous from the standpoint of radiation exposure.

> *. . . . the radiation exposure during a DEXA spine study is the same or less than the radiation exposure to a passenger on a trans-Atlantic airline flight.*

From the medical standpoint, the major advantage of DEXA again involves precision. The refinements made to DEXA are such that small changes in the bone density of 1% to 4% per year can be detected. DEXA has allowed us to expand and refine our knowledge about osteoporosis and quickly determine if a recommended therapy to prevent bone loss is working. DEXA is now considered by most authorities to be the preferred method for measuring the bone mass or, as is commonly said, the procedure of choice.

QUANTITATIVE COMPUTED TOMOGRAPHY (QCT)

Computed tomography or CT scanning (sometimes called "CAT"scans) can also be used to accurately measure the bone density in the spine and other areas of the skeleton. When bone-density measurements are made with computed tomography it is called QCT. This stands for quantitative computed tomography. When QCT is used to measure the wrist or other area in the arms and legs, it is called pQCT. The p stands for peripheral. QCT of the spine does expose the patient to

more radiation than the other techniques and some patients find the test gives them claustrophobia because of the nature of the equipment. Nevertheless, some physicians prefer to use QCT measurements of the spine rather than DPA or DEXA because of its unique ability to measure the very center of the individual bones in the spine, the vertebrae.

Other techniques to measure the bone density and even assess the quality of bone are being developed. Sound waves in the form of ultrasound are being used in medical research to measure both the amount and quality of bone. This technique has been adapted for the knee cap and the heel. It is already in use in Europe. There will undoubtedly be other developments in the future that will improve our ability to measure bone density.

In 1984, the American College of Physicians compared all the techniques to measure bone density that were available at the time. (Since DEXA was not available until 1988, it was not considered in this report.) After comparing the cost, safety, and accuracy of SPA, DPA, and QCT, the American College of Physicians concluded that DPA was the preferred technique. The College has not reconsidered this issue since DEXA became available. As I noted earlier, most authorities feel that DEXA has replaced DPA as the procedure of choice for measuring bone density.

There are several manufacturers of bone-density equipment in the United States. Three of the largest are LUNAR Corp., Norland, and Hologic. All of these manufacturers make excellent machines. DEXA, DPA, and QCT machines are expensive. They are generally too expensive for individual doctors to have in their offices but most major medical centers and some large clinics will have either SPA,

DPA, DEXA, or QCT available. You'll find a list of the major U.S. bone-density equipment manufacturers' telephone numbers in the appendices. If you or your doctor wish to locate a site that provides bone-density testing, a call to the manufacturers can be helpful. The National Osteoporosis Foundation (also see the appendices for more information) may also be able to provide this type of information.

What Do You Have To Do During the Test?

From a patient's point of view, bone-density testing is relatively simple. The tests (SPA, DPA, DEXA, or QCT) are all absolutely painless. There are no pills to take and certainly no injections. You can eat before you go, although it is not generally wise to take a calcium pill that day. This is because the intestinal tract lies on top of the spine and an undigested calcium pill might be measured along with the calcium in the bones. One of the nice things about bone-density testing is that, most of the time, you don't even have to undress. For a DPA or DEXA spine or hip study, you lie on a flat padded table. For an SPA,

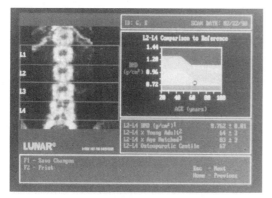

A DEXA bone density report.

DEXA, or pQCT study of the wrist, you sit in a chair.

What Kind of Information Will You Get?

The information a bone-density study provides cannot be obtained in any other way at the present time.

Look at the sample report from a DEXA study of the spine. On the left is the image of the spine which is created by the computer during the test. Although this is a computer image, it is very much like the picture obtained during a regular X ray of the spine. Using this image, the physician identifies each individual bone or vertebra in the spine. The computer measures the size of the vertebra and calculates the amount of mineral in each square centimeter of bone. This is the bone mineral density, or BMD. Usually, an average BMD of three or four vertebrae, rather than one from a single vertebra, is used to make medical determinations. In the sample, the average BMD of the second, third, and fourth lumbar vertebrae has been selected and is highlighted under the graph on the right. This is the L2-4 BMD. The L stands for lumbar. The lumbar spine is the lower part of the spine. It begins at or just slightly above waist level. This area of the spine is examined because it can be measured separately from other parts of the skeleton. A DEXA machine is designed to look straight through the body. There are no other bones that lie in front or behind the lumbar spine. In contrast, the thoracic spine, which begins at the base of the neck and ends at about waist level, has the breastbone (sternum) and ribs in front of it. This currently makes it impossible to measure the thoracic spine without interference from the ribs and breastbone. This is not a disadvantage. In diseases like osteoporosis, the thoracic spine and lumbar spine are equally affected, so it is possible to look at one area of the spine and know what is happening in another area.

Once the L2-4 BMD has been calculated by the computer, two comparisons can be made. The first is called the Young Adult comparison. This compares your measured bone density today with the average bone density of a 30-year-old and computes the results in a percentage. For example, in the report shown, the measured L2-4 BMD was 0.762 g/cm^2. The Young Adult comparison is 64%. This means that this 65-year-old woman, whose bone density today is 0.762 g/cm^2, has a bone density that is 64% of the average 30-year-old woman's. If the assumption is made that this woman had an average bone density when she was 30, the test suggests that she has lost 36% of her bone density. How you compare to the 30-year-old is also used to classify your bone density as normal, osteopenic, or osteoporotic. The World Health Organization published definitions for these terms in 1994, which are based on how far below the young adult bone density your value may be.

The next comparison is the Age-Matched comparison. It is simply a means of comparing your bone density with what is expected for your age. As noted in chapter 1, there is a tendency for both men and women to lose bone density as they grow older. Although we don't consider this to be the result of any kind of disease, it is not desirable. Since we expect you to lose bone with age, you will want to be better than we predict you will be on the basis of the Age-Matched comparison. For the same 65-year-old woman, the Age-Matched comparison was 83%. This means that her measured bone density of 0.762 g/cm^2 is 83% of what we would have predicted if

all we knew about her was her age. Knowing how you compare with your peers is useful to your doctor because an especially low value suggests an unknown cause of bone loss that must be found through a careful medical evaluation.

The most important value on the bone-density test is the measured bone mineral density. The BMD itself is the factor that determines your risk of having a fracture. Once this value is known, it is possible for your doctor to predict what your risk of having an osteoporotic fracture is today or 20 years from now. In general, for each decline in bone density of about 10%, your risk of having an osteoporotic fracture doubles in comparison to the woman who still has the bone density of the 30-year-old.

In the early years of bone-density testing, there was controversy as to whether a woman's risk of developing an osteoporotic fracture could really be predicted from a bone-density measurement. This controversy was often widely publicized. Many doctors hesitated to use bone-density measurements until the controversy was resolved. There is no longer any controversy. There are medical studies of over 20 years in duration that unequivocally show that a woman's risk of having a fracture can be predicted with a bone-density measurement. In fact, a bone density measurement can predict your risk of having an osteoporotic fracture as well as a measurement of blood pressure can predict your risk of having a stroke and even better than a cholesterol measurement can predict your risk of heart disease.

> *. . . a woman's risk of having an osteoporotic fracture can be predicted with a bone-density measurement.*

In the case of the 65-year-old woman, her risk of having an osteoporotic fracture today is increased by 290% compared with the individual who still has the bone density of the average 20-year-old. We can also predict that, without proper intervention, she will experience five osteoporotic fractures in her lifetime. But a little knowledge is a lot of power. With this kind of knowledge, the patient's physician can advise her on how to prevent that from happening. Your physician can do the same for you.

WHEN DO YOU NEED A BONE-DENSITY TEST?

One of the most important medical decisions women must make is whether to take estrogen replacement at menopause. While there are many reasons to take estrogen replacement, one of the most important and uncontroversial is the prevention of osteoporosis. If you are unsure whether you wish to take estrogen, a bone-density measurement will help to determine whether you need estrogen to reduce your risk of osteoporotic fracture. If you have been on estrogen replacement and are considering stopping estrogen, again, a bone-density measurement to determine your risk of having a fracture without estrogen should be done before your decision is made.

We also use bone-density measurements to determine whether the dose of estrogen is sufficient to protect the bones. This is not a universally accepted use of bone-density measurements at this time, but many doctors consider it to be a reasonable approach. The smallest or minimum effective dose of the different estrogen preparations that are FDA approved for the prevention of osteoporosis are known (see chapter 4) but that does not mean that this dose is effective for every woman. With a bone-density test before starting estrogen replacement and then with a second study about a year later, we can be sure that your bones are protected.

Other uses for bone-density measurements have been recommended by the National Osteoporosis Foundation. If your doctor suspects bone loss after performing a regular X ray of the skeleton, the National Osteoporosis Foundation recommends that a bone-density test be done to measure the bone density. Individuals who must take cortisone or similar medications have a high risk of bone loss and the NOF suggests using bone-density measurements to detect this undesirable side effect so that the treatment can be changed.

The average cost of a bone-density test in the United States is $150.00.

If you are going to have a bone-density test, which area of the skeleton should be measured? Most authorities believe that a woman entering menopause who needs this information to help decide whether estrogen replacement is needed for the prevention of osteoporosis should have both the spine and hip measured. Of necessity then, this means that the test must be done on a DPA or DEXA machine. (The ability to look at the hip with QCT is limited.) If DPA or DEXA is not available, a QCT measurement of the spine or an SPA or pQCT measurement of the wrist or heel can be done to make a reasonable assessment of a woman's risk of having a fracture. In other situations, the physician must determine which area of the skeleton is the best to measure with a bone-density test.

WHAT DOES BONE-DENSITY TESTING COST?

The average cost of a bone-density test in the United States is $150.00. Generally, a single photon study of the wrist is the least expensive type of test. DPA and DEXA studies of the spine and hip are usually comparable in price, although DEXA may be a little more expensive. A bone-density study using computed tomography, or QCT, is generally the most expensive. Medicare will cover bone-density testing with DEXA and QCT as well as SPA, but coverage is not available for bone-density testing performed with DPA. In my opinion, there is no good rationale for the lack of Medicare coverage for DPA testing, but it is the case. Many private insurers are beginning to offer coverage for bone-density testing. In fact, several states have passed laws requiring private insurers to offer this type of coverage. You will need to contact your insurance carrier to determine if coverage is available to you for bone-density testing. Reimbursement for the costs of testing may be offered in some circumstances and not in others. Often coverage is not provided if the testing is performed as part of a preventive medicine examination.

Is bone-density testing worth the cost? A survey of California women who had undergone bone-density testing and paid at least $100.00 of their own money found that 83% thought so. An analysis of the costs of treating osteoporosis compared with the costs of bone-density testing at menopause and estrogen replacement to prevent osteoporosis in women whom the test identified as being at risk found that there would be a minimum savings of $27.6 million dollars every year to our economy. But in the end, you must decide for yourself. How much is it worth to know if you are at risk for a spine or hip fracture from osteoporosis so that you can take all the steps necessary to prevent it?

CHAPTER 13

Salmon Calcitonin in the Treatment of Osteoporosis

Many people, including physicians, have never heard of salmon calcitonin. This is somewhat surprising when you realize that salmon calcitonin was approved for the treatment of osteoporosis in 1985 and until late 1995 was one of only two medications approved by the Food and Drug Administration for this purpose. The introduction of nasal spray calcitonin in August 1995, however, has made many people take notice.

Calcitonin is a hormone. Our bodies make calcitonin in the thyroid gland. This isn't the hormone we call thyroid hormone; it is simply made in the same place in the body. Calcitonin's most important effects are on the bones and the way the intestinal tract, blood, bones, and kidneys handle calcium. The body has a marvelous system of checks and balances for all of the different organ systems. The hormone calcitonin is part of the checks and balances system for calcium. If the calcium level in the blood goes up, calcitonin's task is to return the calcium level to normal. It does this by preventing the movement of calcium from the bone to the blood. Calcitonin also may increase the amount of calcium passed into the urine through the kidneys and may decrease the amount of calcium we absorb from the intestinal tract. Calcitonin sounds so much like calcium because it was named for its ability to lower the level of calcium in the blood.

Calcitonin was actually discovered over 30 years ago by a researcher named Dr. D.H. Copp. As research on this hormone continued, it was discovered that human beings were not the only species to make calcitonin. Pigs, eels, sheep, and salmon, to name a few, also made calcitonin. In the United States, laboratory versions of human and salmon calcitonin are used to treat disease.

Human calcitonin is used in the treatment of another bone disease called Paget's disease, which is quite different from osteoporosis. At present, Ciba Pharmaceutical Company markets synthetic human calcitonin under the trade name of Ciba-Calcin. Although this form of calcitonin has been used in research studies on osteoporosis, it is not approved by the FDA for use in the treatment of osteoporosis in the United States. Synthetic human calcitonin is FDA-approved for use in the treatment of Paget's Disease. Synthetic salmon calcitonin can be used for this as well.

Two U.S. pharmaceutical companies make synthetic salmon calcitonin: Rhone-Poulenc Rorer Pharmaceuticals markets an injectable form called Calcimar, and Sandoz Pharmaceuticals makes both an injectable form and the new nasal spray, which are both sold under the name of Miacalcin. Both

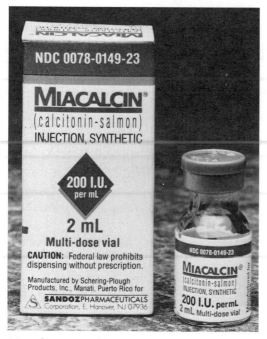

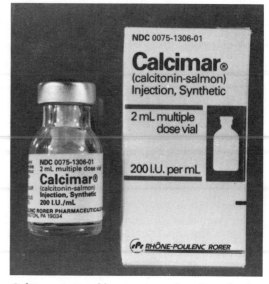

Calcimar Injectable, a registered trademark of Rhone-Poulenc Rorer.

Miacalcin Injectable. Photo courtesy of Sandoz Pharmaceuticals, East Hanover, New Jersey.

Calcimar and Miacalcin are available by prescription only.

Although we believe that calcitonin in human beings is part of the intricate control mechanism for calcium, no one has yet been able to prove that calcitonin deficiency causes osteoporosis. It is clear, however, that treating people who have osteoporosis with salmon calcitonin can be extremely beneficial. Calcitonin can stop bone loss, relieve pain from fractured bones, and may actually stimulate the formation of new bone. Research also suggests that treatment with salmon calcitonin can prevent the development of new fractures caused by osteoporosis.

Calcitonin can stop bone loss, relieve pain from fractured bones, and may actually stimulate the formation of new bone.

How does calcitonin work? We think that the hormone prevents the osteoclasts, the cells that tear down old bone, from functioning. This prevents the loss of bone and the movement of calcium from the old bone into the bloodstream. Exactly how calcitonin prevents the function of osteoclasts is still somewhat theoretical, but it is believed that calcitonin attaches, or binds, to the osteoclast. The ability of the osteoclast to secrete substances that cause bone loss is impaired and the life span of the osteoclast is shortened. Calcitonin may also prevent new osteoclasts from being formed. The result of all this is that bone loss is reduced or halted.

Calcitonin's ability to relieve pain is well known among physicians who have used the drug to treat patients with painful osteoporotic fractures. The mechanism by which calcitonin accomplishes this is again somewhat theoretical, but researchers speculate that calcitonin stimulates the production of the body's own natural pain killers, called endorphins. The inhibition of the osteoclasts may have some pain-relieving benefit in and of itself. There are many reports in the medical literature describing calcitonin's ability to relieve pain from osteoporotic fractures. Most of these reports are what we call anecdotal. That is, they describe what the physician observed and what the patient reported. There are research studies in which women who had experienced osteoporotic spine fractures received either salmon calcitonin or a placebo in order to determine scientifically if calcitonin could really relieve pain. As you can imagine, it is difficult to ask a woman in pain to participate in a research study in which she might receive only a placebo. So, by design, most of these studies are short in duration and do not involve large numbers of women. These studies have consistently shown a marked decrease in pain in the women receiving calcitonin. In one such study, women who had suffered painful spinal fractures were treated with either salmon calcitonin or a placebo within 15 days of the fractures. The women who received calcitonin had a significant reduction in pain within 2 weeks while the women who received a placebo did not show similar improvement for 4 weeks. In another study, women who had suffered a spine fracture within the preceding 3 days were given either salmon calcitonin or a placebo for 14 days. All of the women in this study were also given free access to oral pain medication. By day 3 of the study, the women receiving calcitonin could sit up in bed. By day 4, these same women could stand and were beginning to walk. The women who received placebos remained in bed for the entire 14 days of the study because their pain was too severe to allow them to get up. After the seventh day of the study, the women who received calcitonin did not request any additional pain medication while the women receiving a placebo continued to need additional oral pain medication through the end of the study. Although we expect pain to gradually decline after a fracture as the normal healing process takes place, it is apparent that salmon calcitonin provided quicker pain relief than could be attributed to simple healing.

It is important to note that calcitonin is not an addicting pain medication. It does not cause drowsiness or impair the senses. For patients who are in pain from a recent osteoporotic fracture, calcitonin therapy can reduce their pain so that they need less of the potentially addicting medications and can get back on their feet more quickly. In addition to being able to care for themselves sooner, returning to their feet in less time also means less bone loss from the inactivity will occur, which would only make their osteoporosis worse.

There is also some evidence that patients treated with calcitonin gain new bone, although calcitonin's major effect would appear to be in preventing bone loss. In one research study in women with postmenopausal osteoporosis, 12 months of treatment with salmon calcitonin resulted in a 13% increase in the bone content in the forearm. In another study, there was an 8.5% increase in the spine after 12 months. Perhaps most important, there is evidence that calcitonin treatment helps prevent additional fractures from occurring. In 1992, doctors from Spain reported that a group of women treated with salmon calcitonin for 2 years appeared to be protected from new osteoporotic fractures when compared to a group of women who were not treated. The number of new fractures that occurred in the women treated with calcitonin declined by 60% at the end of 2 years and the number of new fractures in the untreated group actually increased by 35% over the same period of time.

If salmon calcitonin can do all these things, you might reasonably ask why you have never heard of it before and why every woman who developed osteoporosis in the past wasn't prescribed it. There were two major reasons. First, it was expensive, and second, salmon calcitonin was available only as an injection.

INJECTABLE SALMON CALCITONIN

Prior to late summer 1995, the only form of salmon calcitonin that physicians in the United States could use was an injection. Although other forms of salmon calcitonin were in use in Europe and South and Central America, it was not until August 19, 1995, that the FDA approved nasal spray salmon calcitonin for use in the United States.

Injectable salmon calcitonin is still available for use. Standard therapy for osteoporosis with injectable preparations of Calcimar or Miacalcin calls for a daily injection of 100 Units (I.U.). Because the injections are daily, it is impractical for an individual to go to a doctor's office every day to receive his or her injection. This means that patients must learn to give themselves the injection or a family member or friend must help them. It's not difficult to learn to do. Both companies that make salmon calcitonin provide take-home video tapes and written materials on how to give the injections.

The injections are not painful. I use small syringes with very short, small needles. Insulin syringes work very well, but you cannot use the insulin unit marks on the syringe because insulin units and calcitonin units are not the same. The volume markings on insulin syringes can be used to measure the very small amount of calcitonin required for the injections. The

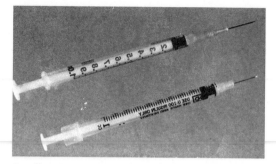

Small syringes are used to administer salmon calcitonin in the treatment of osteoporosis. The needles are only ½-inch long.

medication is injected into the fat underneath the skin, not into the muscle as are other injections you may remember receiving in the past. I have most of my patients start their injections in the top of the thigh because it's an easy area to use. You can see exactly what you're doing and it seems to cause less anxiety when you are just beginning. Different areas of the body can be used for the injections (see the illustration), many of which are quite similar to sites that a diabetic might use for insulin injections.

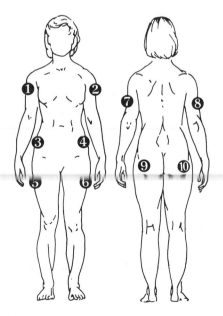

The injection sites

The injections are small. The amount of liquid is at most, $1/10$ of a teaspoon. A little dexterity is required to learn how to draw the medication out of the bottle into the syringe. Actually, I think that is the most difficult part for people to learn. I always show my patients how to do it. I will watch them prepare the syringe and supervise their first injection. I send them home with the videotapes and written materials and then have them return in a week for a second supervised session. I've not had a patient yet who could not learn how to do this, regardless of her age.

The expense of the injectable medication is, in my opinion, the major reason for its limited use. One small bottle of salmon calcitonin will provide four injections of 100 I.U. The cost of one bottle currently ranges from $23 to $32, then there's also the cost of the syringes and cotton and alcohol to cleanse the skin. Recently a decrease in the cost of salmon calcitonin has been the trend. Rhone-Poulenc Rorer and Sandoz periodically offer rebates and discounts to patients to help defray the cost. The wholesale costs to pharmacies have also come down. Some physicians are using lower doses of the injectable salmon calcitonin or giving the medication every other day or only 10 days each month. These approaches, when successful, bring down the cost of treatment with injectable salmon calcitonin.

Injectable salmon calcitonin is a safe medication. The most serious potential side effect is an allergic reaction. In reality, this is quite rare. I always have my patients undergo a skin test before they start the treatment to be sure that they are not allergic to it. The skin test takes only 15 minutes to do. A small amount of a dilute mixture of calcitonin is injected into the skin on the arm. After 15 minutes, if the patient is allergic to the calcitonin, the appearance of the skin will change. Once the skin test is passed, there are no really serious side effects of salmon calcitonin. But there are side effects that can be a nuisance. In about 15% of people, salmon calcitonin therapy will initially cause nausea. The nausea does not persist; that is, it goes away as you continue the treatment. The nausea does not usually progress to vomiting. Some physicians have recommended giving calcitonin at bedtime so that a patient will sleep through any nausea. Others have their patients take a mild anti-nausea medication before their injection. These are reasonable things to do. Remember though, 85% of the time patients don't have any nausea.

The other side effect that also occurs about 15% of the time is a sensation of warmth in the head, neck, and chest. For women, this feeling is like a hot flash. This sensation doesn't last very long and is transient. It goes away as the therapy continues. Again, 85% of the time, this doesn't happen.

A few people will notice an increase in the number of times they have to urinate with calcitonin treatment. This isn't very common at all and has not proved to be a problem.

MIACALCIN NASAL SPRAY

On August 18, 1995, Miacalcin nasal spray, the synthetic salmon calcitonin nasal spray manufactured by Sandoz Pharmaceuticals, was approved by the Food and Drug Administration for the treatment of osteoporosis.

Salmon calcitonin is rapidly absorbed through the tissues in the nose. The medication reaches its highest levels in the blood stream within 30 to 40 minutes. Food, calcium supplements, liquids, or other medications do not affect your ability to absorb salmon calcitonin through the nose as they might some orally administered medications. Other medications do not interact with salmon calcitonin in any significant way at all so you need not worry if it is safe to take other medications if your doctor prescribes salmon calcitonin. The nasal spray can be used any time of day.

All medications that are administered by nasal spray can produce some irritation of the nose itself. Salmon calcitonin nasal spray is no different in this regard. Overall, most individuals can use salmon calcitonin nasal spray with little or no difficulty. In five different research studies that involved a total of 551 women between the ages of 47 and 75, only 3.1% of the women being treated with nasal spray salmon calcitonin stopped treatment because of nasal side effects. The types of nasal side effects that were noted included rhinitis (an irritation of the nose), dryness, itching, nosebleed, and redness. In many cases, these complaints occurred only as a single, isolated event that did not recur even though the women continued to use the nasal spray. In these research studies, about one-fourth of the women treated with Miacalcin nasal spray complained of some type of nasal side effect at least once. Three-fourths of the women had no nasal side effects at all. Smoking did not seem to make nasal side effects any more or less likely. (That doesn't mean it's okay to smoke, of course!) Unlike injectable salmon calcitonin, the nasal spray is much less likely to cause nausea or flushing. Nausea occurs in less than 2% of patients treated with the nasal spray and flushing occurs in less than 1%.

There is a large research study going on now in the United States evaluating the changes in bone density and the risk of fractures in women being treated with Miacalcin nasal spray. This study is intended to last for five years and involves over 1,000 women. We hope to have some preliminary results from this study as soon as it has been underway for a few years. Other smaller studies from Europe are already completed. These studies have consistently shown that Miacalcin nasal spray in a dose of 200 I.U. per day can inhibit bone loss in women who are more than five years postmenopausal. These studies also suggest that Miacalcin nasal spray can reduce the risk of new spine fractures by more than 50%. The final word is expected to come from the large United States research study, but our expectation is that it will confirm these earlier results.

Salmon calcitonin nasal spray, like its injectable cousin, has the ability to relieve the severe pain from osteoporotic fractures. There is information that suggests that the nasal spray can begin to relieve pain even more quickly than injectable calcitonin.

Miacalcin nasal spray comes in a pump spray bottle, not a squeeze spray bottle like decongestant nasal sprays. The bottle should be kept in a regular refrigerator until you are ready to use it. Don't put it in the freezer! Once you have opened it, you can keep the bottle at room temperature. Before you use the sprayer, you must first screw the pump on the bottle and then activate it. You activate the pump by holding the bottle upright and simply depressing the white side arms toward the bottle about six times. You'll see a faint mist come from the nozzle. You do not need to activate the pump before every use. Do this only the first time you use a new bottle. You're now ready to use the sprayer. Just insert the nozzle firmly into the nose while sitting or standing up. Then depress the pump toward the bottle. You don't have to inhale while you do this so you need not worry about jeopardizing your future in politics.

Each spray bottle is intended to last about two weeks with daily use. Each spray delivers the recommended amount of 200 I.U. You should alternate the side of the nose each day. You can use some simple way of remembering which side of the nose you used yesterday. Perhaps even days of the month can be the right side and odd days, the left. If you have been using the injectable salmon calcitonin and are going to change to the nasal spray, there is nothing special that you need to do. You can simply stop the injections one day and begin using the nasal spray the next.

Nasal spray salmon calcitonin is much like its cousin, injectable salmon calcitonin, in that it is effective in retarding

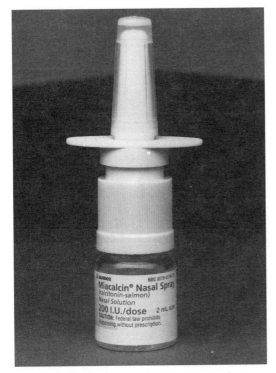

Miacalcin Nasal Spray. Photo courtesy of Sandoz Pharmaceuticals Corporation.

bone loss and reducing fracture pain. I fully expect the United States research studies using nasal spray salmon calcitonin to confirm the results of earlier studies that suggest the nasal spray will also reduce the risk of fractures. Although the nasal spray is obviously administered differently from injectable salmon calcitonin, the drug itself has been in clinical use to treat osteoporosis for eleven years in the United States at this writing, during which its safety has been clearly established. The nasal spray formulation has actually been in use in twelve other countries for up to ten years now. One of the most important differences between the injectable salmon calcitonin and the nasal spray, however, is the cost. The nasal spray, even though a larger dose is required, is much less expensive, costing only about $50 to $55 a month.

Strictly speaking, salmon calcitonin is only approved by the FDA for use in the treatment of osteoporosis. However, it can be used in some circumstances as a preventive measure as well. In a woman who is at high risk for osteoporosis and who cannot take estrogen replacement, salmon calcitonin may be useful. For example, a woman who has had breast cancer is almost always advised not to take estrogen replacement at menopause. If a bone-density test is done and she is found to have a low bone density, her physician might wish to consider salmon calcitonin as a preventive measure. Several research studies have demonstrated that salmon calcitonin can also prevent the bone loss that occurs with estrogen deficiency.

Salmon calcitonin can be a marvelous medication for a woman who is in pain from osteoporosis. One of my favorite patients is a woman in her early eighties who had already had several fractures in her spine before she came to see me. She walked with a cane and was always in pain because of her spine. I talked to her about salmon calcitonin therapy and her initial response was that it seemed too difficult and she thought she was "too old" and "too far gone" to bother. She had become quite depressed because of her situation and because of the medication she was taking to relieve the pain from the fractures. Finally, she reluctantly agreed to try calcitonin.

I taught her how to give herself the injections and counseled her on getting adequate calcium and vitamin D. I also gave her some gentle exercises for her back muscles and started her on a gradual walking program. Her improvement was steady over the next year. Bone-density studies showed an increase in the bone strength in both her spine and hip. Her pain de-creased. As her pain lessened, she became more active. As she became more active, her sense of well-being and purpose improved. Her depression lessened. After 1 year of treatment I received a call from one of her other doctors who said that he initially failed to recognize her when she had come into his office earlier in the day. She looked so much better, he couldn't believe she was the same woman! He wanted to know what miracle I had wrought. It wasn't a miracle. It was salmon calcitonin, calcium, exercise, and a little encouragement from me.

My patient has actually returned to working in her husband's office. She still walks with a cane, but not because she needs it as a walking aid. She uses it as a weapon to move people out of her way!

CHAPTER 14

Alendronate (Fosamax) and Related Drugs in the Treatment of Osteoporosis

You know that nasty soap scum ring around the tub and sink that build up over time, especially if you have hard water? Believe it or not, in developing chemicals that could be added to detergents to prevent the development of soap scum, scientists created a whole family of medications known as the bisphosphonates, some of which are now being used in the treatment of osteoporosis. The bisphosphonates soften hard water by attaching themselves to the minerals in the water. They love calcium! And in the human body they head straight for the bones in order to attach themselves to the mineral in the bone. Once in the bone, they do much more than peacefully reside there. The bisphosphonates inhibit the function of the osteoclasts, the cells that resorb or tear down old bone. The resulting effect is to retard or even stop bone loss.

There are quite a few different members of the bisphosphonate family. They all have similar sounding names ending in "-dronate" like etidronate, alendronate, risedronate, and pamidronate. The grandfather of all the bisphosphonates is etidronate, which has been available by prescription in the United States for some time. Etidronate is sold under the trade name of Didronel and is manufactured by Procter & Gamble Pharmaceuticals. Didronel has not been approved for the treatment of osteoporosis in the United States although it is approved for the treatment of a disease called Paget's Disease. Although Paget's Disease also affects the bone, it is very different from osteoporosis. Didronel has been used in research studies as early as 1976 to treat osteoporosis. The success of this research in large measure helped to spur development and testing of other bisphosphonates, which most of us fondly refer to as "son or grandson of Didronel."

INTERMITTENT CYCLICAL THERAPY OF OSTEOPOROSIS WITH DIDRONEL

The results of two of the most important research studies using Didronel in the treatment of osteoporosis were both published in the *New England Journal of Medicine* in 1990. The first study, from Denmark, involved 66 women whose average age was 68 and who already had at least one fracture in their spine. All of the women were given 500 mg of calcium and 400 units of vitamin D every day. Half of the women received a 400 mg tablet of Didronel daily for 2 weeks only out of every 15 weeks. The other half of the group received a placebo tablet for 2 weeks out of every 15 weeks. This cycle of 2 weeks on, 13 weeks off was repeated 10 times for a total of 150 weeks in the research study. The bone density in the spine was measured at the beginning and end of the study, and the number of new spine fractures that developed was also noted. Because Didronel was given for only 2 weeks out of every 15 weeks, this form of therapy was called intermittent cyclical therapy, or "ICT," with Didronel.

At the end of the 150 weeks, the amount of mineral in the spine had increased 5.3% in the women who received Didronel, while the women who received placebos lost 2.7%. During the second and third years of the study, the women being treated with Didronel had far fewer new spine fractures than the women who were treated with the placebo. There were no serious side effects from the Didronel in this study.

Just a few months after the Denmark study was published, the results of a large study done in the United States was published in the *New England Journal of Medicine*. This study involved 429 women. The women in this study were all at least 1 year past menopause and had to have at least 1 spine fracture. Their average age was 65. The 429 women in this study were actually divided into four different groups; one group received intermittent cyclical therapy with Didronel. At the end of two years in this study, these women had increased the bone density in their spines 4.3%. As in the Denmark study, it also appeared that the women treated with Didronel were much less likely to have a new spine fracture. Side effects of the medication were infrequent and not serious in this study. There were some reports of nausea and diarrhea, but over-

all, the women did not seem to experience any real problems from the use of Didronel when it was given intermittently.

Didronel was not given every day in these research studies because it was known that the daily, long-term use of Didronel could cause the bone to become structurally abnormal. It was thought that intermittent use of the medication would be enough to stop bone loss and reduce the risk of fractures without causing the bone to become abnormal. This appears to be true. Women in both of these studies underwent biopsies of their bones so that the bone could be examined under the microscope. In all cases, the bone was normal.

Didronel can be obtained by prescription and many physicians have prescribed it for their patients with osteoporosis. Nevertheless, Didronel is not approved by the Food and Drug Administration for either the prevention or treatment of osteoporosis. It seems unlikely that Didronel will be approved for this use any time soon. Why?

The research studies using intermittent cyclical Didronel were designed to show whether Didronel increased or preserved the bone density better than calcium alone. This it did. The problem is that the FDA requires that a research study demonstrate convincingly that Didronel would reduce the risk of new fractures. The studies did suggest this, but they weren't "convincing" in statistical terms. As a consequence, Didronel was not approved for the treatment of osteoporosis.

There are other members of the bisphosphonate family that are being tested in research studies now. These medications have names like risedronate, tiludronate, ibandronate, and so on. They differ from Didronel slightly. Most of these drugs are thought to have Didronel's ability to stop bone loss without the risk of causing an abnormal bone. In that sense, they are considered an improvement over Didronel. One of these new bisphosphonates was approved by the FDA for the treatment of osteoporosis on September 25, 1996. The drug is called alendronate and is manufactured and sold by Merck under the trade name of Fosamax. The speed with which Fosamax was approved by the FDA was dramatic. The information from the research studies done in both the United States and Europe was so strong that the FDA moved briskly to approve Fosamax.

FOSAMAX (ALENDRONATE SODIUM) IN THE TREATMENT OF OSTEOPOROSIS

Fosamax is the "son" of Didronel. Its chemical structure is similar in some respects but very different in others. Its ability to stop bone loss is hundreds of times more potent than that of Didronel, and at the same time, it is much less likely to cause the development of an abnormal bone. As a consequence, instead of being given intermittently, Fosamax is given every day. The research study that gained Fosamax FDA approval for prescription use in the treatment of osteoporosis involved almost 1,000 women. The study was done both in the United States and Europe and the results were published in November 1995 in the *New England Journal of Medicine*.

The 994 women who participated in this research study were all postmenopausal women between the ages of 44 and 84. When they began the research study, all of the women had bone densities in the spine that were considered osteoporotic. The study lasted for three years.

At the end of the study, the women who had received 10 mg of Fosamax every day had increased the bone density in their spines by an average of 8%. In the hip, their bone densities had increased by an average of 4.5% to 7%, depending upon the area within the hip that was measured. Even more important was that Fosamax treatment clearly reduced the likelihood that a woman would have an osteoporotic fracture. Although some of the women who were treated with Fosamax during the research study did have a new spine fracture as did some of the women who were given a placebo, the fractures that the women who were treated with Fosamax experienced were fewer in number and less severe.

Fosamax also proved to be very safe. The women in this research study who were given Fosamax had few side effects, and when they did, they were generally minor. Most of the side effects were gastrointestinal in nature, like nausea, diarrhea, or constipation. This is rather typical of this family of medications, not just Fosamax. The likelihood that these things will happen if you take Fosamax is really quite small. Nausea occurs only 3.6% of the time and constipation or diarrhea only 3.1% of the time. So overall, 96% to 97% of the time, these things don't happen.

Another characteristic of medications in the bisphosphonate family like Fosamax is that they are poorly absorbed from the stomach when you take them as a pill. Because of this, it is absolutely imperative that you take Fosamax on an empty stomach with a full glass of water. First thing in the morning at least 30 minutes before breakfast is recommended. If there is any food in your stomach, or if you take the medication with coffee or juice instead of water, you won't absorb any of the medication. It is also extremely important that, when you get up in the morning to take Fosamax, that you stay up after taking it. Don't go back to bed and wait for breakfast! Staying up helps to reduce the likelihood that any of the Fosamax would come up from the stomach back into the esophagus (the tube that goes from the mouth to the stomach). Severe irritation of the esophagus can occur if this were to happen—even to the point of causing an ulcer in the esophagus. Fosamax is not recommended for individuals who have kidney failure. Those individuals would not be able to eliminate the medication from their bodies properly. It is also not recommended for individuals who have serious gastrointestinal problems to start with. There does not seem to be any problem with taking other medications along with Fosamax, although they should not be put in the stomach at the same time.

Fosamax comes in two different doses, but only one of the doses is used to treat osteoporosis. The recommended dose for the treatment of osteoporosis is one 10 mg tablet taken once a day. There is a 40 mg tablet, but this is used for the treatment of Paget's Disease. Fosamax is available only by prescription. A month's worth will generally cost around $50, although prices will certainly vary from pharmacy to pharmacy. Fosamax was approved by the FDA for the treatment of osteoporosis on September 25, 1995. Of all of the FDA-approved treatments that we currently have for osteoporosis, it is the only non-hormonal preparation available in tablet form. Fosamax is a welcome addition to the battle against osteoporosis.

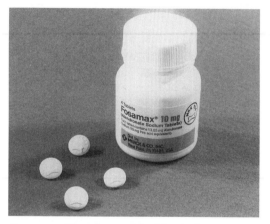

Fosamax. Manufactured by Merck & Company. Photo courtesy of D. McBee, Media Services, Texas Woman's University, Denton, Texas.

CHAPTER 15

Future Therapies for Osteoporosis

Conjugated equine estrogen (Premarin), salmon calcitonin (Calcimar or Miacalcin), and alendronate (Fosamax) are the only forms of treatment that are FDA approved at present. Although all three of these therapies are effective, they are not suitable for everyone who develops osteoporosis. The only FDA-approved medication for the prevention of osteoporosis is estrogen. But there are women who cannot take estrogen replacement at menopause because of other medical problems. We need other options to offer people, other alternatives to estrogen, calcitonin, and alendronate.

The nature of research is such that the development of new medications proceeds slowly. Research is underway for some of these options, exploring the possibilities of new drugs and new uses for existing drugs.

Much interest is currently centered around seven types of medications: sodium fluoride, bisphosphonates, designer estrogens, thiazide diuretics, calcitriol, androgens, and the flavanoids. In fact, a special kind of sodium fluoride is being considered for approval by the FDA now.

SODIUM FLUORIDE

As explained in chapter 10, a disease known as fluorosis was noted many years ago in miners and industrial workers who were exposed to fluoride dust. They in-haled the dust and the dust coated their skin. The individuals who developed fluorosis complained of pain in the bones and were noted to break bones more easily. Yet when their bones were X rayed, they appeared to be extremely white on the X rays, indicating an increase in their thickness or density. In other words, these people had an increased amount of bone as a result of their exposure to fluoride, but the bone had become abnormal.

Out of the recognition of this disease came the realization that fluoride could in some way stimulate the formation of new bone. Researchers hoped they could harness this ability and control it so that new bone made under the influence of fluoride would be healthy and strong.

This research is proceeding. At present, it is clear that when sodium fluoride is given in tablet form in an amount of 50 mg or more a day, most patients will respond with an increase in bone of as much as 10% per year in the spine. Fluoride appears to do this by increasing the number of osteoblasts, the cells in the bone responsible for bone formation.

In spite of the gains seen in bone density, the early research using regular forms of sodium fluoride caused us to question whether the new bone made in the spine was strong bone. After all, our goal is to prevent fractures. It serves no purpose at all to increase the amount of bone if the new bone is weak or abnormal. In research studies in which fluoride has been given to women with osteoporosis, the most important outcome of the study is whether the number of new fractures the women suffer during the study is reduced by the treatment. If the women treated with fluoride have measurable increases in the amount of bone in the spine and have fewer spinal fractures when compared to a similar group of women who were not treated with fluoride, researchers confidently conclude that the new bone is strong bone. In some studies, researchers will also biopsy the bone in women who have been treated with fluoride to see if the bone appears normal under the microscope.

Some studies have shown that women treated with regular sodium fluoride have fewer fractures than women who were not treated. Other studies could show no difference. In a recent large study at the Mayo Clinic, women were treated with a fairly large dose of sodium fluoride for 4 years. Although they gained almost 9% in their spinal bone density every year during each of the 4 years, they had almost as many fractures as a group of women in the study who were not treated with fluoride. It appeared that the new bone was not strong bone after all.

Although dramatic gains in bone density in the spine have been seen with regular sodium fluoride, it remained unclear what the fluoride was doing to the bone density in the hip. Some research studies found that the bone in the hip decreased with fluoride treatment while other studies did not. And finally, there was serious concern about the side effects of regular sodium fluoride therapy. Regular fluoride can wreak havoc with the stomach. Nausea, vomiting, pain, bleeding, and even ulcers have been reported with fluoride treatment. Individuals treated with fluoride can also develop a painful

condition called plantar fasciitis. This refers to pain in the arch of the foot caused by inflammation of the tissues that make up the arch. The pain can be a mild nuisance or so distressing that it prevents an individual from walking.

Although the Mayo Clinic study was important, it was not considered the final word. Many authorities felt that the dose of regular sodium fluoride the Mayo Clinic used was too large. Other studies using smaller doses of fluoride have resulted in gains in spinal bone density and apparent protection from fractures. Some researchers also believe that fluoride therapy must be interrupted periodically in order to allow the new bone to form properly. And finally, some researchers have turned to different preparations of sodium fluoride in order to minimize the side effects and better control the amount of fluoride in the bloodstream.

Dr. Charles Pak and his colleagues at the University of Texas Southwestern Medical School in Dallas, Texas, have developed a new kind of sodium fluoride called slow-release sodium fluoride. It is this new kind of fluoride that has been recently considered for approval by the FDA for the treatment of osteoporosis.

Slow-release sodium fluoride is a tablet that is specially formulated to allow small amounts of fluoride to be released at a time into the intestinal tract. Avoiding large amounts of fluoride in the stomach at one time dramatically reduced the likelihood of the stomach problems that had been seen with regular fluoride. The carefully controlled release of medication from the tablet also allowed Dr. Pak to control the amount of fluoride circulating in the bloodstream. In two different research studies, which were published by Dr. Pak and his colleagues in 1995, postmenopausal women with osteoporosis were treated with slow-release sodium fluoride in a dose of 25 mg twice a day. They also received calcium citrate supplements. The women benefited from gains in bone density in the spine without experiencing any loss of bone density in the hip. They also reduced their risk of future spine fractures and experienced far fewer side effects than previously seen with other forms of fluoride. After reviewing Dr. Pak's research, an FDA advisory committee recommended that slow-release sodium fluoride be approved for the treatment of osteoporosis. The full FDA, however, declined to approve slow-release sodium fluoride, wanting to see more research on this promising drug.

Because sodium fluoride is a stimulator of new bone formation, slow-release sodium fluoride would be an exciting addition to our weapons in the treatment of osteoporosis. It is likely to be several more years, however, before the drug is approved.

OTHER BISPHOSPHONATES

In Chapter 14, we discussed the original bisphosphonate called etidronate, or Didronel, and the new bisphosphonate alendronate, or Fosamax, which was approved in September 1995 for the treatment of osteoporosis. But there are several other bisphosphonates that are being evaluated to prevent or treat osteoporosis in research studies. They all have similar sounding names, ending in "-dronate." These are medications like pamidronate, ibandronate, tiludronate, and risedronate. Pamidronate is already available by prescription under the name of Aredia. This medication is not taken orally. It is given intravenously and used to treat abnormally high levels of calcium in the blood,

which might be seen with certain types of cancer. There was a tablet form of pamidronate that was used briefly in research studies to treat osteoporosis, but it was found to cause severe irritation in the esophagus and stomach. As a consequence, the tablet form of pamidronate is no longer available. Other bisphosphonates have shown a great deal more promise in the prevention or treatment of osteoporosis when given in tablet form. One of the other interesting characteristics of the bisphosphonate family is that they seem to help prevent the spread of breast cancer to the bone. If this can be conclusively proven in research studies, the bisphosphonates would become an even more desirable choice of treatment for the woman who has had breast cancer who cannot take estrogen.

DESIGNER ESTROGENS

I really don't like this phrase to describe this new class of medications, but it is the slang description that is being used to describe medications that act like estrogen but which are not really estrogen at all. The goal here is to develop a medication that will do all of the good things that estrogen can do without doing any of the bad. For example, we would like an estrogenlike medication to prevent bone loss without causing menstrual-like bleeding and endometrial cancer and without affecting the breasts. We would also like such a drug to lower cholesterol, keep the skin healthy, and stop hot flashes, too. Sound too good to be true? Well, there's certainly no harm in trying, and that's exactly what researchers are trying to do.

One of the most promising drugs in this category is a medication called tibolone. This is a medication that is made entirely in the laboratory. It is not estrogen at all, but it acts primarily like estrogen in the human body. It also acts a little bit like progesterone and a very little bit like testosterone (which is okay because women are supposed to have a little testosterone). Tibolone is not new. There is information in the medical literature on tibolone and its effects that dates back over 20 years. Interest in tibolone, however, has dramatically increased in the last few years. Research studies have shown that most women who take tibolone do not have any menstrual bleeding, and there is no proof to date that tibolone will cause endometrial cancer. At the same time, tibolone appears to stop bone loss, stop hot flashes, lower total cholesterol, and help improve a woman's overall quality of life. Research studies using tibolone are going on now in the United States in order to give our FDA sufficient information so that it can be considered for prescription use here. Tibolone is already available in Europe for women to use and is sold by prescription there under the trade name of Livial.

There is another totally different group of "designer estrogens" that act like estrogen in some parts of the body and not in others. One of the first of these was actually tamoxifen, which is now being used to prevent the recurrence of breast cancer. Tamoxifen seems to act like estrogen when it comes to the bones, so it helps to prevent bone loss. It also acts like estrogen in the uterus, so it can stimulate the tissues in the uterus that may lead to the development of endometrial cancer. But when it comes to the breasts, it is an anti-estrogen. This type of drug, which acts like estrogen in some tissues and is an anti-estrogen in others, is called an estrogen agonist/antagonist.

Tamoxifen is not used to prevent or treat osteoporosis, although it may certainly help to protect a woman who has had breast cancer who cannot take estrogen for osteoporosis. Other drugs in this class are being tested to see if they would be useful in preventing osteoporosis. Their names sound somewhat similar. These are drugs like droloxifene and raloxifene. Raloxifene, which is made by Eli Lilly, appears to inhibit bone loss and reduce cholesterol without stimulating the breast or uterine tissue. Droloxifene, made by Pfizer, also seems to have the beneficial effects of estrogen on bone and cholesterol without the undesirable effects on the uterus or breast. It will be exciting to see what information will be learned in the next few years about these "designer estrogens."

THIAZIDE DIURETICS

Thiazides are a type of diuretic. You may be more familiar with the term fluid pill than diuretic. This type of medication is often prescribed to reduce swelling in the legs or to lower blood pressure. A diuretic causes the kidneys to increase the amount of water and sodium lost into the urine each day. The natural side effect is having to go to the bathroom more often. There are many different chemical types of diuretics. Thiazide diuretics are one chemical type. There are many different brands of thiazide diuretics. Some of the names under which they are sold by prescription only include Diuril, Enduron, Esidrix, HydroDiuril, and Oretic. Aldactazide, Maxzide, and Dyazide contain thiazide diuretics in addition to another ingredient. There are other brands as well, too numerous to name.

In 1990 in the *New England Journal of Medicine,* doctors reported that men and women 65 years of age or older who were taking thiazide diuretics were found to have a lower risk of hip fracture than men and women of similar age who did not take thiazide diuretics. These men and women were given prescriptions for thiazide diuretics primarily to control high blood pressure. They were not being used to prevent osteoporosis. The risk of hip fracture in the thiazide-treated group was about two-thirds that of the group not taking the thiazides. In 1991, another group of physicians reported similar findings. How could a diuretic protect an individual from hip fractures?

Although thiazide diuretics increase the amount of water and sodium lost from the body into the urine each day, they actually decrease the amount of calcium lost into the urine. In other words, they have the ability to help the body conserve calcium. By reducing the amount of calcium lost every day, they reduce or prevent calcium deficiency. That should benefit the bones. In fact, as early as 1983 it was reported that individuals who used thiazide diuretics had an increased bone density compared with those who did not use thiazides.

This promising evaluation was contradicted in late 1991 in the *Annals of Internal Medicine* by a report that said thiazide diuretics did not protect individuals from hip fracture at all. In this same report, it was also noted that another non-thiazide type of diuretic called furosemide actually increased an individual's risk of hip fracture. In this case, the doctors theorized that by lowering the blood pressure the diuretics could make people light-headed when they stood up and increase the likelihood of falling. Furosemide is a different type of diuretic than the thiazides. Is it generally considered more potent and does not help the body retain calcium. In fact, in some circumstances furosemide can actually increase the amount of calcium lost in the urine. It is true that any kind of diuretic can cause the blood pressure to drop if the individual is sensitive to the drug or if the dose is too high.

The report did dampen our enthusiasm for using thiazides to prevent or treat osteoporosis. In May of 1993, a group of researchers decided to specifically evaluate whether thiazides increase a woman's risk of falling and whether they have any effect at all on her risk of having a fracture. They found that women who had used thiazides for at least 10 years had a greater bone mass than women who had not used thiazides. In addition, the women taking the medication did not fall any more often than women who were not taking thiazides. Finally, women taking thiazides had a slightly lower risk of hip and wrist fractures than women not taking thiazides although the reduction in risk was not dramatic.

What does all this mean? At present, most physicians limit the use of thiazide diuretics in the prevention or treatment of osteoporosis to the patient who is losing abnormally large amounts of calcium into the urine every day. In this situation, the thiazide will reduce the amount of calcium being lost. In individuals who have a normal amount of calcium in the urine and who do not have another reason—like high blood pressure—to need a thiazide diuretic, there is not yet enough hard evidence that a thiazide diuretic would really be beneficial.

Thiazides, like all diuretics, have their own side effects. Excessive water loss can occur, leading to dehydration. Potassium and magnesium are lost from the body along with sodium, also as a result of taking a diuretic. The loss of potassium and magnesium can have serious consequences. In addition, thiazide diuretics may have an undesirable effect on cholesterol and blood sugar levels. Some diuretics are worse in this regard than others. So, like any other drug used in medicine, the potential to do good must outweigh the potential to do harm before a drug should be prescribed. More research is needed before thiazide diuretics should be used as a general preventive measure for osteoporosis or as part of the treatment of every patient with osteoporosis.

THE FLAVANOIDS

The flavanoids are chemical compounds that are really quite common and yet most people are not aware of their existence. Flavanoids are found in plants and there are probably over 4,000 different kinds. In fact, we eat about a gram of flavanoids every day. In the 1930s, scientists discovered that some of the different flavanoids had vitaminlike properties. Flavanoids have been the mainstay of folk remedies for many years to treat thyroid and other hormone-related problems. Some of the flavanoids have been found to have anticancer properties, which has created a great deal of interest and excitement. You have probably already realized that flavanoids may also have an effect on the bone.

In 1985, reports began appearing on the ability of a synthetic flavanoid called ipriflavone to have a beneficial effect in osteoporosis. Ipriflavone seems to have the ability to block bone loss and may also stimulate bone formation. How ipriflavone works is still somewhat speculative. So far the drug's side effects have

been relatively minor. There is still a lot to be learned about the flavanoids, but this area has exciting potential in the treatment of osteoporosis as well as other diseases.

ANDROGENS

Androgens refer to hormones that have similar properties to the male sex hormone testosterone. Testosterone itself has been used in osteoporosis, not only in men, but in women as well. Research has also focused on synthetic, testosteronelike substances, called anabolic steroids.

Nandrolone decanoate is an anabolic steroid that is given by injection. Several research studies have demonstrated that women treated with nandrolone increased their calcium absorption and bone density in their spines and forearms. This type of therapy has not been viewed with a great deal of enthusiasm because of the possibility of virilizing side effects such as increased hair growth or deepening of the voice. While those side effects do occur, they have tended to be less severe than initially feared.

Testosterone itself can be found combined with estrogen in pills that are available in the United States. Women normally make testosterone in the ovaries and adrenal glands. Although this amount of testosterone is small in comparison to the amount of testosterone a man has, it may still be very important to a woman's well-being. Physicians have recognized for some time that when a woman must have her ovaries removed surgically, even though she is given estrogen replacement, she may not regain her sense of well-being, energy, or sex drive unless a small amount of testosterone is included with her estrogen replacement. Research is now being conducted to see if testosterone replacement in addition to estrogen replacement in these woman might result in better protection from osteoporosis.

CALCITRIOL

Calcitriol is the name for the form of vitamin D that is made in the kidney. The actual chemical name for calcitriol is 1,25 dihydroxy-vitamin D. Calcitriol is available in pill form and is sold by prescription under the trade name of Rocaltrol, a registered trademark of Roche Laboratories.

Calcitriol is the most potent form of vitamin D available. Researchers became interested in calcitriol as a possible treatment for osteoporosis when it was realized that there might be a connection between the declining production of calcitriol by the kidneys in older women and the development of osteoporosis. Older women with osteoporosis have been found to have lower levels of calcitriol than women who do not have osteoporosis. Low calcitriol levels would cause poor absorption of dietary calcium in the intestines leading to calcium deficiency.

It is also now known that calcitriol can have a direct effect on the bone. Calcitriol may actually stimulate both the bone-forming osteoblasts as well as the bone-resorbing osteoclasts. As you can imagine, we would like to improve calcium absorption and stimulate the osteoblasts to make bone without stimulating the osteoclasts to cause bone loss. One additional concern is that because calcitriol is so potent, too much calcitriol can cause the level of calcium in the blood and urine to go too high, both of which can have serious consequences.

The research is promising but far from complete. Studies have demonstrated that calcitriol can increase calcium absorp-

tion and increase the bone mass in the spine and forearm. High calcium levels in the blood and urine have developed in some patients, requiring investigators to carefully control the amount of calcium in the diet or lower the dose of calcitriol. It remains to be seen whether several years of calcitriol treatment can be safely undertaken and if protection from fractures results from this type of treatment.

THE FUTURE

The future looks very bright. In addition to the seven medications or types of medications listed here, there are perhaps 30 more medications that have the potential to be useful in treating or preventing osteoporosis. As a physician, I eagerly anticipate the development of some of these new therapies. As women, you and I can't afford to wait for the future to begin preventing osteoporosis. Getting adequate calcium, exercise, and vitamin D; avoiding cigarette smoke and excessive alcohol; and, for some, taking estrogen replacement at menopause, will successfully prevent the majority of osteoporosis that exists now. All of these measures, as well as salmon calcitonin or alendronate can be used to effectively treat osteoporosis. Our options will almost certainly increase in the next decade but we have effective options now—we just need to take advantage of them.

CHAPTER 16

Osteoporosis in Men

Osteoporosis does affect men, but not to the same extent it affects women. The differences between men and women, which seem to protect men from osteoporosis, are worth studying because they give us clues about how women can protect themselves from osteoporosis. Even though osteoporosis is correctly viewed as largely a woman's disease, men do need to recognize that they can develop osteoporosis and take the necessary steps to protect themselves.

When researchers began studying various populations to look at the quantities of different types of fractures that occurred in men and women and when they occurred, it readily became apparent that there were significant differences between us. In childhood and young adulthood, boys and men have more fractures of the arms and legs than women. From around the age of 35 and until age 70 or so, the number of limb fractures experienced by men drops off dramatically. After the age of 70, the number of fractures begins to rise again. In contrast, young girls have far fewer arm and leg fractures than young boys. Similarly, young women have fewer fractures than young men. But around the age of 45, there is an abrupt increase in the number of women's limb fractures that continues to rise sharply as the women grow older.

It isn't too difficult to understand why boys break more arms and legs than little girls when one looks at the types of activities the two groups have traditionally participated in. With contact sports and the generally more vigorous physical play that boys engage in, there is greater opportunity for broken bones to occur. But why do men experience a second rise in fractures, primarily in the hip, late in life? This rise is similar to the increase in hip fractures that occurs in women, but it happens later and never reaches the same magnitude.

Another interesting trend appeared when researchers looked at spinal and wrist fractures in men and women. The number of spinal fractures begins to increase sharply in women around the age of 55 and continues to increase as the women grow older. Spinal fractures in men are relatively uncommon at any age. Wrist fractures also increase in women around the age of 45 or 50. Wrist fractures in men are relatively uncommon and do not seem to increase in number at any particular time during mature adult life. Again, why is this?

What do we have in common that would cause both men and women to have hip fractures late in life? And why do men have far fewer hip fractures than women? What is so very different between men and women that men do not have the spinal and wrist fractures that women have?

What we have in common is calcium deficiency. What separates us is the amount of bone we develop as youngsters and the female menopause.

Peak bone mass, or the maximum bone density that a young individual reaches by the end of his or her third decade of life, is clearly different between men and women. Although men are taller than women on average and therefore could be said to have more bone overall, the density or strength of that bone is not determined by an individual's height. But men, on average, have a peak bone mass that is 25% to 30% greater than a woman's. This greater peak bone mass means that any bone loss that may follow is beginning from a much higher level of bone strength. More bone will have to be lost before the bone becomes fragile enough to break than if the bone loss had begun from a lower overall level. All other things being equal, the occurrence of fractures will be delayed in time.

As we know, a significant portion of peak bone mass is determined by inheritance. Good nutrition and exercise also influence how dense the bones become. Good nutrition for the bones means adequate calcium. While most girls become calcium deficient around the age of 15 because they eliminate beverage milk from their diets, boys do not stop drinking milk until around the age of 25. One can only speculate why this occurs. Perhaps girls and women become concerned about their weight and calorie intake in the adolescent years and decide milk is a caloric beverage easily eliminated from the diet.

Regardless of the reasons, milk is eliminated from the diet and replaced with low- or no-calorie, noncalcium-containing beverages like soda, tea, or coffee. Boys and men continue to drink milk longer. Again, one can only speculate that boys and young men may continue to drink milk into young adulthood because of its association with athletic prowess and fitness. That 10-year difference in milk consumption and adequate dietary calcium may be a critical element in a man's ability to develop a greater peak bone mass than a woman's.

Another factor in the development of peak bone mass is the level of physical activity. The children and young adults that are more physically active will develop a greater peak bone mass. In our society it has traditionally been the young boy or man who participates in organized physical activities and sports. This has also contributed to the development of a greater peak bone mass in men. Fortunately, social acceptance for organized physical activities and sports for girls and women has increased in recent years. This will benefit those young women in later life.

After the age of 25, men become calcium deficient as well. However, men still tend to consume a greater number of calories per day overall and this means that they will obtain a greater amount of calcium from nondairy sources than women, who consume fewer calories. As a consequence, their calcium deficiency is never as great as women's. Men have also remained more physically active as mature adults. So while men experience bone loss as a result of calcium deficiency, this loss is taken from a higher level of bone due to their greater intake of calcium and increased level of exercise as young boys and men.

The bone loss men experience proceeds at a much slower rate than that of a woman's. This slower rate is again due to a less severe calcium deficiency and a greater level of physical activity. Men lose about 0.3% of their bone per year after the age of 40 from areas of the skeleton like the hip. Women lose about 0.8% per year, or more than two and one-half times more. The calcium deficiency we have in common would appear to be instrumental in causing hip fractures in both men and women. The man's greater peak bone mass and slower rate of calcium-deficient bone loss offers him greater protection and, as a result, fewer hip fractures occur in men.

Spinal and wrist fractures have one thing in common. They involve areas of the skeleton that are predominantly composed of a type of bone known as trabecular bone. In contrast, the hip is predominantly composed of a type of bone known as cortical bone. Spinal and wrist fractures, fractures in trabecular bone, are common in women with osteoporosis but not in men. The explanation here would appear to be that sex hormone deficiency accelerates the loss of trabecular bone that ultimately leads to fractures.

Sex hormone deficiency is expected in women. The failure of the ovaries that causes estrogen deficiency occurs in every woman at menopause around age 50. Men do not have a similar "male menopause," or a period when their testosterone levels are expected to abruptly fall. Testosterone levels do decline gradually as a man ages. There is speculation that this gradual decline may contribute to some bone loss in men but the effects are much less dramatic than the loss of bone in women caused by a woman's menopause. The amount of bone men lose from the spine and wrist over a lifetime is much less than what women lose. Women may lose as much as 47% of their bone density from the spine and 39% from the wrist over their lifetime. Men, on the other hand, lose only about 14% from both. As a result, men do not experience the osteoporotic wrist and spinal fractures that are so tragically common in women. Men who have suffered diseases like mumps (which can affect the production of testosterone by the testes) after reaching adulthood can and do develop spinal fractures. Other diseases like pituitary tumors and alcoholism can also cause testosterone levels to decline. If testosterone is not replaced, loss of bone will occur, much as it does in women when a woman's estrogen levels fall.

All of the diseases that can cause or contribute to osteoporosis in women can also affect men. The medications that have been noted to cause bone loss in women will also cause bone loss in men. We both experience some decline in the function of the bone-forming cells as we age, which leads to less bone being formed. But because of men's greater peak bone mass, slower rate of bone loss, and the absence of an expected "male menopause," they have generally been protected from the ravages of osteoporosis. Only $1/6$ to $1/7$ of all osteoporotic spinal fractures occur in men. Only $1/4$ to $1/5$ of all hip fractures occur in men.

Men should not be lulled into a false sense of security because osteoporosis is not as common in them as in women. The risk of a man developing an osteoporotic hip fracture in his lifetime is about 17%. Osteoporotic hip fractures kill men just as surely as they kill women. The risk of developing other types of osteoporotic fractures is less, but certainly should not be ignored.

In one study from Wisconsin, out of 114 men over the age of 65 who had no history of injury to the back, 13 were found to have wedge compression fractures in the spine. That's 11% of the men in the study.

To prevent osteoporosis in men, correction of dietary calcium deficiency is important, just as it is for women. Although the RDA for calcium, according to the National Osteoporosis Foundation, is 1,000 mg for men after the age of 24, this may not be ideal. Dr. Jeffrey Jackson, an expert on osteoporosis in men at Scott and White Clinic and Texas A&M School of Medicine, recommends that men over the age of 55 consume 1,500 mg a day and increase their vitamin D intake to a total of 600 to 800 units a day. Important also is

---

RISK FACTORS FOR OSTEOPOROSIS IN MEN

Caucasian ancestry | Lean body build
Sedentary lifestyle | Testosterone deficiency
Alcoholism | Cigarette smoking
Calcium deficiency | Some gastrointestinal surgery
Cortisone use | Excess thyroid hormone replacement

---

the early recognition of testosterone deficiency. Men are often hesitant to complain of declining sexual function or decreased libido, even to their physicians. Testosterone replacement is available in injections, pills, and even a testosterone patch (much like the estrogen patch for women). A simple blood test that measures the level of testosterone and a pituitary hormone called LH can determine if there is a problem that requires testosterone replacement.

There are recognized risk factors for osteoporosis in men just as there are for women. In a study from the Mayo Clinic, researchers found a strong association between cigarette smoking and alcohol consumption and the development of osteoporosis in men, suggesting that these habits cause bone loss in men. A study from the University of Indiana also found an association between smoking and alcohol consumption and bone loss in men.

AN OSTEOPOROSIS PREVENTION PLAN FOR MEN

1. Meet the Recommended Daily Allowance for Calcium!

Boys and men between the ages of 11 and 24 need 1,200 mg to 1,500 mg a day. Between the ages of 25 and 65, the amount recommended by the National Institutes of Health is 1,000 mg a day. After the age of 65, the NIH recommends 1,500 mg a day for men, just as they do for postmenopausal women not taking estrogen and all women over 65.

2. Obtain adequate Vitamin D.

Fifteen minutes of sunshine exposure per day is generally adequate for this purpose. If this is not possible, a good multivitamin that provides 400 units of vitamin D is desirable. After the age of 65, multivitamin supplementation with 400 units of vitamin D is generally recommended.

3. Keep up a lifelong exercise program.

Incorporate elements of aerobic weight-bearing exercise and strength training into a regular exercise program.

4. Don't smoke.

5. Avoid daily alcohol consumption and drink in moderation.

6. Report any loss of sexual function or desire to your physician.

7. Ask your doctor if any of the medications you must take or any of the surgery that you may have had could increase your risk of osteoporosis so that preventive measures can be taken.

The 50 Most Commonly Asked Questions

1. **Isn't osteoporosis just part of growing old?**

No, no, no, no. It is true that osteoporosis was once thought to be the inevitable consequence of growing older, particularly for women. We now know osteoporosis is a *disease*. When you realize that it is a disease, with specific causes, you realize that it can be prevented and treated.

2. **Why do women develop the hump in the back with osteoporosis?**

In medical terms, the hump is called kyphosis. In lay terms, it is called a dowager's hump or widow's hump. It is the result of a change in the curve in the spine that is caused by the occurrence of multiple fractures in the individual bones of the spine or vertebra. This should not be confused with the small hump that both men and women can develop at the base of the neck and upper back. This is a fat pad, which can become very prominent with weight gain. This has a name, too. It's called a buffalo hump. It is not at all related to osteoporosis.

3. **Is it true that women become shorter when they develop osteoporosis?**

A woman can lose height as the result of osteoporosis. The loss of height results from the fracture or collapse of the bones of the spine. This loss of height is permanent and can be as much as 5 or 6 inches.

4. **Why do women get osteoporosis more often than men?**

Men do develop osteoporosis. But men tend to develop a greater bone density as children and young adults because they participate in physical activities more often and their calcium intake tends to be more sufficient. This greater bone mass helps to protect them. Also, men do not experience an abrupt decline in midlife in their sex hormone, testosterone. All women experience menopause, which causes estrogen levels to decline dramatically. This loss of the female sex hormone causes a marked loss of bone in many individuals. If men had a similar male menopause in which testosterone was abruptly lost, we would see more osteoporosis in men.

5. **Women didn't develop osteoporosis as often in the nineteenth century. Why?**

Fortunately or unfortunately, women did not live long enough in the nineteenth century to develop osteoporosis. For the average woman, menopause signaled not only the end of her ability to have children but also the end of her life. Now women are living a full third of their lives after menopause and there is more than enough time to develop osteoporosis.

6. **Is it ever too late to benefit from calcium?**

No. For the child, adequate calcium helps to develop a greater bone mass. For the mature adult, adequate calcium helps to maintain the bone mass. Even in the very old, calcium supplementation to meet the RDA can halt the bone loss that is due to calcium deficiency. Even though some bone may have already been lost, stopping this loss and providing stability to the bones is of value in preventing fractures.

7. Can you get too much calcium?

Yes, but it is difficult to do unless one takes far too many calcium supplements. While it is beneficial for every individual to meet his or her RDA for calcium, there is no proven benefit to exceeding the RDA. Calcium intakes of 3,000 or 4,000 mg a day may provide more calcium than the kidneys can remove from the body and may result in a kidney stone. Any individual who has had a kidney stone in the past should consult his or her physician before increasing his or her calcium intake (even to the RDA). Certainly, if an individual has been advised to avoid calcium-containing foods, a physician should be consulted.

8. Is it better to get calcium from the diet or from supplements?

There is no dependable information at this point to say that diet is better than supplements or that supplements are better than diet. The important thing is to meet your RDA for calcium. If you elect to use dairy products as your calcium source, you should certainly use low-fat dairy products.

9. Should you take your calcium supplement at night?

The time of day is not important. It is desirable to spread your calcium sources out over the day. Some supplements are more effective when taken with food and some should be taken on an empty stomach. Careful reading of the label is important.

10. Do calcium supplements have any side effects?

The most common side effects of calcium carbonate supplements are gas and constipation. Calcium citrate seems to cause much less trouble in this regard. Most people can take these supplements without difficulty but individual sensitivities do vary.

11. Does it make any difference if you drink whole milk as opposed to skim milk?

Skim milk is certainly better for you because it eliminates unnecessary milk fat. Skim milk actually has a little more calcium than whole milk, so you certainly don't lose any of the bone benefits by drinking skim milk.

12. I have pain in my back. Could that be osteoporosis?

Osteoporosis generally does not cause pain until a bone actually breaks. Fractures in the spine are visible on regular back X rays. Your doctor can evaluate you for this possibility. In the absence of a fracture, the pain is most likely caused by any one of several problems that are unrelated to osteoporosis and can affect the back.

13. Does osteoporosis run in families?

Yes, it would appear so. Most researchers think that what is inherited is not a tendency to lose bone as an adult but a tendency to make less bone as a young individual. This makes the development of osteoporosis more likely later on.

14. My grandmother broke her hip, but the doctor didn't call it osteoporosis. Was it osteoporosis?

It may have been. Remember that osteoporosis was not considered a disease in your grandmother's time. It was often simply considered part of the aging process. As a result, many women who had broken bones were not told that they had osteoporosis. The physician would not consider it important to tell the older woman that she had developed another "sign of old age."

15. Will I have any warning that I am developing osteoporosis?

Not in terms of the way you feel. The loss of bone is silent. A woman can feel perfectly well today and have a spinal or hip fracture tomorrow from osteoporosis.

16. How can I know for sure if I am at risk of developing osteoporosis?

Only one test can accurately measure the bone strength and predict your risk of having a fracture. That test is called bone densitometry.

17. What are the best types of exercise for me to do?

From the standpoint of bone health, weight-bearing and strength-training exercises are the best. Although swimming is an excellent cardiovascular exercise, it is not a good bone exercise. Bicycling is also not the best bone exercise. While walking is a weight-bearing exercise, you will need to walk briskly, at least 3 mph and preferably 4 mph, to get the bone benefit.

18. Won't I look like the weight lifters on TV if I do strength-training exercises?

No, you don't have to lift those kinds of weights to get the bone benefit. But you will find that as the muscles and skin tone up with the exercise, you'll have a much more attractive figure as well as better bones.

19. Does every woman need estrogen to protect her from osteoporosis?

No. Some women develop a bone mass that is so good prior to menopause that simply meeting their calcium needs and exercising regularly can protect them. But there is no way for you to know without a bone-density test.

20. How much does a bone-density test cost?

Prices vary certainly. The national average is $150.00.

21. Is the radiation from a bone-density test dangerous?

The newer techniques like dual photon absorptiometry and dual energy X-ray absorptiometry deliver a very small amount of radiation, which is not dangerous. In fact, the amount of radiation from a dual energy X-ray measurement of the spine's bone density is very similar to the amount of radiation an individual receives when flying across the Atlantic on a commercial airliner!

22. Is osteoarthritis the same thing as osteoporosis?

No. Osteoarthritis is a disease in which the lining of the joints becomes inflamed. This produces pain and can ultimately destroy the joint. This is quite different from osteoporosis in which mineral is lost from the bone itself, leaving the bone more easily broken. It is, unfortunately, quite possible for an individual to have both osteoarthritis and osteoporosis.

23. Do you need to take a vitamin D supplement in order to benefit from calcium?

Vitamin D is necessary for the body to properly utilize the calcium you eat in the diet or get from a supplement. Vitamin D is made in the skin from exposure to the sun. Most individuals under the age of 60 do not need extra vitamin D unless they get no sun exposure. After the age of 60 a supplement may be wise. The vitamin D does not need to be taken at the same time as the calcium-containing food or calcium supplement. In certain circumstances, your doctor may advise measuring the vitamin D level in your blood to see if you need a prescription form of vitamin D.

24. Are scoliosis and osteoporosis related?

Scoliosis refers to a condition in which the spine develops an S curve. The spine may also rotate abnormally in scoliosis. Scoliosis can occur in growing youngsters and can also develop in older adults. It is considered to be a totally separate disease from osteoporosis. However, it has been noted that many women who have osteoporosis also have scoliosis. While this does not prove that one disease causes the other, the association is worrisome.

25. Can certain medications cause osteoporosis?

Yes. Unfortunately, some medications can be extraordinarily beneficial and at the same time cause bone loss that can lead to osteoporosis. Some of the most important medications are cortisone and prednisone, thyroid hormone, dilantin, lasix, cyclosporin, and lithium. If you are taking any of these medications, don't stop them on your own! Talk to your doctor about what you should do to prevent osteoporosis.

26. Does smoking increase the risk of osteoporosis?

Yes. Smoking actually affects a woman's estrogen levels and ovaries. Smoking causes estrogen to be changed in the liver into a different form that is less beneficial in protecting the bones. Also, women who smoke become menopausal earlier than women who do not smoke.

27. Can coffee really cause osteoporosis?

It's not the coffee that's the problem. It's the caffeine. Excessive caffeine actually causes the body to lose more calcium every day through the kidneys into the urine. Caffeine from any source, whether it's coffee, tea, or cola-based soft drinks, can contribute to this. It's wise to limit your caffeinated beverages to no more than two per day. Then drink decaffeinated.

28. Once you have osteoporosis, can anything really be done?

Yes, definitely. There are effective treatments, even for women who have already suffered fractures from osteoporosis and are in pain. Salmon calcitonin, as either an injection or a nasal spray, is approved by the FDA for the treatment of osteoporosis. Estrogen replacement, often thought of as a means of preventing osteoporosis, is also an effective treatment. Alendronate (Fosamax) is the most recent addition to the FDA-approved therapies for osteoporosis. Slow-release sodium fluoride may also be available in the future to treat this disease. Adequate calcium and vitamin D, along with carefully structured exercise programs, can all be combined with prescription therapies to successfully relieve pain, increase strength, halt bone loss, and reduce the risk of future fractures.

29. Don't I need to take magnesium as well as calcium?

Magnesium is also a mineral, like calcium. But it is called a trace mineral because we need so little. It is very unusual for an otherwise healthy individual to need supplemental magnesium because the little we need is readily available from the diet. The most common exception is the individual who must regularly take a diuretic, or fluid pill. This type of medication can cause magnesium loss. If you are taking diuretics, you should discuss this with your doctor.

30. If my doctor prescribed estrogen replacement to prevent osteoporosis, how long do I have to take it?

Assuming that you became menopausal around the age of 50, most authorities feel that estrogen should be continued for at least 10 to 15 years to prevent osteoporosis. This decision should really be made on an individual basis rather than arbitrarily deciding in advance how long to take it. When I prescribe estrogen for a patient to prevent osteoporosis, I view it as a lifelong commitment unless a problem develops that requires me to stop estrogen replacement. You should not stop estrogen replacement for any reason without consulting your physician.

31. Doesn't estrogen cause breast cancer?

The honest answer is that we don't think so, but we really don't know. Many good researchers are trying to find the answer to this very troubling question. There are two schools of thought at present. One school of thought is that estrogen does not cause cancer, but it may promote the growth of a preexisting cancer. The second school of thought is that there may be an increased risk of cancer from estrogen replacement, but the increase in risk is small and occurs after 10 to 15 years of use. The best advice at this time is to have a mammogram before starting estrogen, do monthly breast self-examinations, and have regular checkups and periodic mammograms.

32. Is it true that estrogen replacement is of no benefit in preventing osteoporosis unless it is started within 3 years of menopause?

No. The longer one waits to start estrogen replacement, the greater the amount of bone that may have already been lost. But estrogen replacement will stop the bone loss caused by estrogen deficiency no matter when it is started.

33. What is the average age of menopause?

Interestingly, the average age of menopause has not changed much over the course of recorded medical history. The average age is 50 to 51.

34. How can I know if I am becoming menopausal?

The approach of menopause is often signaled by the onset of hot flashes. The periods generally become irregular before completely stopping. At first, they may be closer together than usual and then, finally, farther apart. If a woman has had a hysterectomy (the surgical removal of the uterus) and has not had the ovaries removed as well, it may be difficult for her to know when she has become menopausal. Laboratory tests ordered by a physician can clarify this when necessary. If a woman undergoes the surgical removal of both ovaries, she is immediately menopausal.

35. If I take estrogen replacement and the second hormone progesterone, and I begin menstruating again, can I become pregnant?

You will not become pregnant because of the estrogen and progesterone you are taking. How-

ever, most authorities recommend some type of continued contraception, if desired, for at least 1 year after the onset of a nonsurgical menopause because the ovaries can resume intermittent function during this time.

36. I am using a vaginal estrogen cream. Is this enough to protect me from osteoporosis?

Some of the estrogen from the vaginal cream is absorbed into the bloodstream. But the small amount that is required to prevent dryness in the vagina may not be enough to protect the bones from osteoporosis.

37. I am taking an estrogen tablet, but it is not one of the brands that you said were approved by the Food and Drug Administration to prevent osteoporosis. Does this mean that it's illegal or that it won't work?

No. It is certainly not illegal. And it does not mean that it will not work. It simply means that the FDA has not been provided with research for that specific brand that shows it will prevent osteoporosis.

38. I was told that my blood calcium level was high. Does that mean I should stay away from dairy products and calcium tablets?

The level of calcium in the blood is very carefully regulated by the body. If the level is high, a thorough medical evaluation is in order to determine the cause. Rarely does the amount of calcium consumed in the diet cause the level of calcium in the blood to be too high.

39. If my blood calcium level is normal, does that mean I don't have osteoporosis?

Unfortunately, no. The level of calcium in the blood is expected to be normal, even in advanced cases of osteoporosis. The calcium in the bones will be low, but that is not indicated by the blood measurement.

40. What is the vinegar test for calcium supplements?

This is a test to see if the tablet disintegrates properly under conditions that are intended to mimic the conditions in your stomach. Drop a calcium tablet into a glass of vinegar that is at room temperature. Stir vigorously for 30 minutes. The tablet should have disintegrated into fine particles at the end of that time. If it did not, it probably won't disintegrate in your stomach either.

41. What dose of estrogen should I take if I need it to prevent osteoporosis?

There is no one single dose of any estrogen product that is right for every woman. We do know the minimum effective dose of the different estrogen products that have been approved by the FDA for the prevention of osteoporosis. The doses are: Premarin, 0.625 mg; Estraderm™ (estradiol transdermal system), 0.05 mg; Estrace, 0.5 mg; and Ogen, 0.625 mg. These doses are determined by studying large groups of women. The doses listed above are the average doses that were effective. Since it is an average, it means that some women needed less and some women actually needed more. These doses are the starting doses.

42. If I have a bone-density test to determine my risk for osteoporosis, which one should I have?

This is a mildly controversial area in the field of bone densitometry. There are people who strongly favor one type of testing over another for a variety of different reasons. My own preference is to use dual energy X-ray absorptiometry, or DEXA, to measure the spine and hip to determine a woman's risk for osteoporosis. However, it is reassuring to note that there is very good research showing that virtually any of the different techniques like SPA, DPA, and QCT—along with DEXA—can be used to measure the various areas of the skeleton and predict a woman's future risk of osteoporosis.

43. Do I need to have a bone-density test every year?

No. Most authorities recommend having a bone-density test done at menopause to help determine if you need estrogen to protect your bones. A test should also be done if your doctor suspects bone loss after seeing a regular X ray. Testing at other times is generally done on the specific recommendation of your physician. If you are being treated for osteoporosis, a bone-density test may be done yearly to monitor the progress of your treatment. But from a preventive medicine standpoint, bone-density testing is generally needed only two or three times at most during a woman's lifetime.

44. My mother has osteoporosis and is in pain. Is there any treatment that might help her?

Yes, unquestionably. There is a medication called salmon calcitonin, which is available as either an injection or as a nasal spray. The injectable form was approved by the FDA in 1985 for the treatment of osteoporosis. The nasal spray was approved in August 1995. Salmon calcitonin has the potential to stop bone loss, relieve the pain from fractures, and reduce the risk of future fractures. Both forms of salmon calcitonin require a prescription. Injectable salmon calcitonin is sold under the trade name of Calcimar, which is made by Rhone-Poulenc Rorer, or the name Miacalcin, which is made by Sandoz. The regimen that is recommended for injectable salmon calcitonin is 100 I.U. every day, although other regimens may be used. Sandoz's Miacalcin is also available as a nasal spray. The recommended dose of the nasal spray is 200 units a day. Calcium, vitamin D, and exercise are also beneficial. Estrogen has been shown to be worthwhile in the treatment of osteoporosis in women up to the age of 80. Alendronate, or Fosamax, is also available for the treatment of osteoporosis. While all of these medications are useful in preventing bone loss and reducing the risk of fractures, only salmon calcitonin offers the added benefit of pain relief.

45. I've read that boron will prevent osteoporosis. Is that true?

Boron is a mineral that is found in bone. There are only a very few research studies involving a small number of people that have examined the effects of either boron deficiency or boron treatment on osteoporosis. It is much too premature to recommend taking boron as a treatment or preventive measure for osteoporosis. Excessive boron can be toxic. The small amount of boron found in standard multivitamin plus mineral combinations is safe. I do not recommend specific boron supplements at present.

46. I exercise regularly, get plenty of calcium, don't smoke, don't drink alcohol, and there is no osteoporosis in my family. Can't I just continue as I am without worrying about osteoporosis at menopause?

I wish you could, but the truth is that you cannot assume that you will be protected. You should certainly continue to exercise, get your RDA for calcium, and avoid cigarette smoke. This will be of benefit to you. Estrogen deficiency at menopause, however, can be so overwhelming to the bones that calcium and exercise may not be enough to protect them. A bone-density test is the only way at present to determine what is happening to the bones. You can use the information you get from a bone-density test to help you decide if you need estrogen replacement to protect the bones.

47. I've read that fluoride in drinking water can prevent osteoporosis. I've also read that fluoride can cause osteoporosis. Are either of these statements true?

There isn't a simple yes or no for this question. Fluoride is a mineral that is often added to drinking water to help prevent dental cavities. Fluoride has also been used in much larger amounts than are found in water to treat osteo-

porosis. Fluoride can stimulate the bone-forming cells, called osteoblasts, to make more bone, at least in the spine. Some research studies suggested, however, that in areas of the country where the amount of fluoride in the water was high, more people broke their hips than expected. And so questions have been raised about fluoride's effects on the bone in the hip. Questions have also been raised about the bone in the spine, because early studies using fluoride to treat osteoporosis could not prove that the risk of fracture decreased in spite of gains in bone density in the spine. This suggested that the bone was not structurally normal. Recent research done by scientists at the University of Texas Southwestern Medical School using a new form of fluoride called slow-release sodium fluoride has demonstrated fluoride's ability to reduce the risk of spine fracture while increasing the bone in the spine with no apparent harm to the hip. In addition, this form of fluoride appears to have far fewer side effects than earlier forms of fluoride, which could be devastating to the stomach. Slow-release sodium fluoride was recommended for approval by an FDA advisory committee to treat osteoporosis but the full FDA did not approve it. Research in this area is continuing.

48. Can I take estrogen and Fosamax or estrogen and salmon calcitonin together?

Each of these medications by itself has been shown to be effective in treating osteoporosis. The real question is can you combine them and do better than if you took only one by itself? We don't know. There are two published medical studies, one of which looked at the combination of estrogen and calcitonin and the other at the combination of estrogen and etidronate, a drug similar but certainly not identical to Fosamax. Both of these studies suggested that the combinations were better than either one alone in increasing the bone density. Nevertheless, the studies involved a relatively small number of women and are not considered the final say in this matter. In addition, it is not clear that better gains in bone density necessarily means a greater reduction in the risk of osteoporotic fractures. It makes sense that it would, but this certainly has not been proven. There are research studies underway now looking at this very question. At the moment, these combinations are not universally recommended.

49. What is ADFR therapy for osteoporosis?

The initials ADFR do not stand for any particular medication. They actually stand for the sequence of events that we try to create during treatment with any one of several different medications. "A" stands for activate. During the "activation period" a medication is given that stimulates the osteoblasts, which make new bone, and the osteoclasts, which remove old bone. "D" stands for depress. During this period a medication is given that will "depress" the bone-losing cells, the osteoclasts. "F" can stand for either "free" or "formation." During this period no medication is given or a medication that will directly stimulate the bone-forming osteoblasts is given. Finally, "R" stands for repeat. This whole sequence is started all over again. With ADFR, we are trying to artificially manipulate the bone to get the maximum gain in bone along with the maximum suppression of bone loss. Various combinations of medications are used in ADFR

therapy. In some research studies it has been very successful. Since multiple drugs are used in this regimen, it can be a little complicated and each drug used has its own potential for side effects. ADFR therapy is also called coherence therapy.

50. Why are we hearing so much about osteoporosis now? Is this a new disease?

In a sense, osteoporosis is a disease of the twentieth century. In the nineteenth century, the average woman died within 5 years of menopause. She did not live long enough to develop osteoporosis. Now, a woman who reaches the age of 50, the average age at which menopause occurs on the average, can expect to live into her eighties. There is more than enough time for osteoporosis to develop. As this disease has become more common, there has been greater interest among physicians and researchers. We also had to wait for advances in technology like bone densitometry to begin to study the causes of bone loss and to study those treatments that we believed would stop bone loss. In addition, because this is predominantly an older woman's disease, society had to recognize that the health of older women is important. We, as women, had to begin to demand better health care. All of these things, both scientific and social, have come together to bring osteoporosis into the public eye.

Calcium Supplements by Type

This list of supplements was compiled by surveying a private pharmacy, a major grocery store chain pharmacy, and a major drugstore chain pharmacy. This list is provided for informational purposes only. Each product should be carefully examined for the amount of elemental calcium per tablet and documentation on the packaging that indicates that the product passes USP dissolution and disintegration standards. (Inclusion on this list is not intended as an endorsement of the product.)

Calcium Citrate
  Citracal
  Citracal Caplets + D
  Citracal Liquitab
  NutraVescent Calcium Drink
  Windmill Calcium Citrate

Calcium Carbonate
  Calcium-Rich Rolaids*
  Calel-D
  Caltrate 600
  Caltrate 600 + Vitamin D
  Extra-Strength Rolaids*
  Jameson Calcium 600
  Jameson Calcium 600 with Vitamin D
  Jameson High Potency Natural Oyster Shell
    Calcium
  Liqui-Cal
  Nature Made 100% Natural Oyster Shell
    Calcium with Vitamin D
  Nature Made 100% Natural Oyster Shell
    Calcium Extra Strength
  Os-Cal 500
  Os-Cal 500 Chewable
  Os-Cal 250 + D
  Os-Cal 500 + D

  Scientific Nutrition Calcium 600
  Top Care Calcium
  Top Care Calcium Hi-Cal
  Tums
  Tums EX
  Windmill Oyster Shell Calcium
    + Vitamin D
  Windmill Oyster Shell Calcium
  Your Life Natural Oyster Shell Calcium

Calcium Phosphate, Dibasic
  Dical-D

Calcium Phosphate, Tribasic
  Posture
  Posture + D

Mixed Calcium Gluconate, Lactate, and Carbonate
  Calcet
  Fosfree

*Note: Regular, Original, Spearmint, and Wintergreen Rolaids *do not* contain calcium carbonate. Extra-Strength, Cherry, and Peppermint Rolaids can be used as a calcium carbonate supplement.

Common Calcium Supplements

This list of supplements was compiled based on a survey of a private pharmacy, large grocery store chain pharmacy, and large drugstore chain pharmacy. This list is provided for informational purposes only. (No endorsement of any product is implied by inclusion on this list.)

Brand Name	Type of Salt	Made By	Mg/Tab.*	Vitamin D Units	Take with Meals
Calcet	Mixed	Mission	152.8	100	Yes
Calcium-Rich Rolaids**	Carbonate	Warner	220	0	Yes
Calel-D	Carbonate	Rorer	500	0	Yes
Caltrate 600	Carbonate	Lederle	600	0	Yes
Caltrate 600 + Vitamin D	Carbonate	Lederle	600	125	Yes
Citracal	Citrate	Mission	200		No
Citracal Caplets + D	Citrate	Mission	315	200	No
Citracal Liquitab	Citrate	Mission	500		No
Dical-D Tablet	Phosphate	Abbot	117	133	Yes
Dical-D Wafer	Phosphate	Abbot	232	200	Yes
Extra-Strength Rolaids	Carbonate	Warner	400	0	Yes
Fosfree	Mixed	Mission	175.5	150	Yes
Jameson Calcium 600	Carbonate	Jameson	600		Yes
Jameson High-Potency Natural Oyster Shell Calcium	Carbonate	Jameson	500	0	Yes
Jameson Cal 600 with Vitamin D	Carbonate	Jameson	600	125	Yes
Liqui-Cal	Carbonate	Advanced Nutritional	600	0	Yes
NutraVescent Calcium Drink	Citrate	CIMA Labs	500	200	No
Nature Made 100% Natural Oyster Shell Calcium with Vitamin D	Carbonate	Nature Made	500	200	Yes
Nature Made 100% Natural Oyster Shell Calcium Extra Strength	Carbonate	Nature Made	625	0	Yes
Os-Cal 250 + D	Carbonate	Marion	250	125	Yes
Os-Cal 500	Carbonate	Marion	500	0	Yes
Os-Cal 500 Chewable	Carbonate	Marion	500	0	Yes
Os-Cal 500 + D	Carbonate	Marion	500	125	Yes
Posture	Phosphate	Whitehall	600	0	
Posture + D	Phosphate	Whitehall	600	125	
Scientific Nutrition Calcium 600	Carbonate	Mission	600	100	Yes
Top Care Calcium	Carbonate	Topco	600	0	Yes
Top Care Calcium Hi-Cal	Carbonate	Topco	500	0	Yes
Tums	Carbonate	SmithKline	200	0	Yes
Tums EX	Carbonate	SmithKline	300	0	Yes
Windmill Calcium Citrate	Citrate	Windmill	200	0	No
Windmill Oyster Shell Calcium + Vitamin D	Carbonate	Windmill	250	125	Yes
Windmill Oyster Shell Calcium + Vitamin D	Carbonate	Windmill	500	125	Yes
Windmill Oyster Shell Calcium	Carbonate	Windmill	500	0	Yes

*Milligrams of elemental calcium, not total milligrams of calcium salt.

**Note: Regular, Original, Spearmint, and Wintergreen Rolaids *do not* contain calcium carbonate and should not be used as calcium supplements. Extra-Strength, Cherry, and Peppermint Rolaids do contain calcium carbonate and may be used as calcium supplements.

Calcium Content of Common Foods

A quick review of this list will emphasize the importance of dairy products in providing the bulk of our dietary calcium. This list was compiled from a variety of nutritional resources. Calcium content may vary from brand to brand.

Food Group/Food	Serving Size	Calcium in Milligrams
Dairy Products		
MILK		
Whole	1 cup	291
2%	1 cup	297
1%	1 cup	300
Skim	1 cup	302
Buttermilk	1 cup	285
Nonfat, dry	1/4 cup	377
YOGURT		
Low-fat	1 cup	415
Frozen	1 cup	240
Fat-free frozen	1/2 cup	112
CHEESE		
Cheddar	1 ounce	204
Monterey Jack	1 ounce	212
Ricotta, part skim	1/2 cup	337
Parmesan	1 tablespoon	69
Cream cheese	2 tablespoons	23
Muenster	1 ounce	203
Cottage, 2% fat	1/2 cup	78
Mozzarella, skim	1 ounce	207
American	1 ounce	174
Swiss	1 ounce	272
Blue	1 ounce	150
Colby	1 ounce	194
ICE CREAM (11% fat)		
Regular	1 cup	176
Soft Serve	1 cup	236
Seafood		
Sardines, including bones	3 ounces	372
Salmon, including bones	3 ounces	167
Mackerel, canned	3 ounces	205
Oysters	1 cup	226
Tuna	3 ounces	10
Red snapper	3.5 ounces	16
Shrimp, batter-dipped and fried	3.5 ounces	72
Brook trout, cooked	3.5 ounces	218
Vegetables		
Broccoli, fresh cooked	1 cup	136
Turnip greens, fresh cooked	1 cup	252
Collards, fresh cooked	1 cup	357
Green beans, frozen	1/2 cup	31
Lima beans, frozen	1/2 cup	19
Carrot sticks	1 carrot	19
Corn, frozen	1/2 cup	2
Okra, frozen	1/2 cup	88

Calcium Content of Common Foods

Food Group/Food	Serving Size	Calcium in Milligrams
Vegetables		
Green peas	1/2 cup	19
Potato, baked with skin	1 medium	20
Cauliflower, raw	1 cup	25
Celery, raw	1 stalk	20
Onion, raw	1 medium	27
Summer squash, raw	1/2 cup	28
Fruits and Nuts		
Almonds	1/4 cup	94
Brazil	1/4 cup	62
Filberts (hazelnuts)	1/4 cup	54
Peanuts	1/4 cup	21
Apple	1 medium	10
Orange	1 medium	52
Banana	1 medium	7
Pear	1 medium	19
Peach	1 medium	5
Cantaloupe	1/4 medium	14
Grapefruit	1/2 medium	14
Strawberries	1/2 cup	11
Apricots, dried	10 halves	16
Meats/Proteins		
Beef, rib roast	3 ounces	9
Chicken, fried	1 leg	12
Egg, hard boiled	1 large	28
Ham, baked	3 ounces	6
Pork chop	3 ounces	13
T-bone steak	3 ounces	6
Lamb chop	1 chop	4
Sausage, smoked pork	1 link	20
Turkey breast, roasted and without skin	3 1/2 ounces	19
Grains and Breads		
Bagel	1	29
White bread	1 slice	32
Whole-wheat bread	1 slice	20
Cornflakes	1 ounce	1
Rice	1 cup	11
Oatmeal	1/2 cup	10
Crackers, saltine	4 crackers	3
Crackers, graham	2 crackers	6
Dinner roll	1	24
Pancakes, 4-inch diameter	2	72
Waffle, 7-inch diameter	1	179
Spaghetti	1 cup	16
Common Fast Foods		
Arby's Regular Roast Beef Sandwich	1	80
Burger King Whopper	1	100
Jack in the Box Jumbo Jack	1	100
McDonald's Big Mac	1	203
Wendy's Single Burger on White	1	40
Church's Fried Chicken, white meat	3.5 ounces	94
Kentucky Fried Chicken, original	1 breast	50
Taco Bell Taco	1	111
Pizza, 10-inch diameter	1/2	290

Medications that May Affect Your Ability to Exercise

If you are taking any of the medications on this list for any reason, consult your physician before beginning an exercise program. **Do not stop taking any medication without first consulting your doctor.** Taking these medications does not mean that you cannot exercise. You may just need to take certain precautions to ensure that you exercise safely.

Brand Name	Generic Name
BETA BLOCKERS	
Blocadren	Timolol
Cartrol	Carteolol
Corgard	Nadolol
Corzide	Nadolol and Bendroflumethiazide
Inderal	Propanolol
Inderide	Propanolol and Hydrochlorthiazide
Kerlone	Betaxolol
Levatol	Penbutolol
Lopressor	Metoprolol
Sectral	Acebutolol
Tenoretic	Atenolol and Chlorthalidone
Tenormin	Atenolol
Timolide	Timolol and Hydrochlorthiazide
Visken	Pindolol

Beta blockers may slow the heart rate or affect the expected increase in heart rate with exercise.

CALCIUM CHANNEL BLOCKERS	
Adalat	Nifedipine
Calan	Verapamil
Cardene	Nicardipine
Cardizem	Diltiazem
DynaCirc	Isradipine
Isoptin	Verapamil
Nimotop	Nimodipine
Plendil	Felodipine
Procardia	Nifedipine
Vascor	Bepridil

Calcium channel blockers can slow the heart rate and cause some light-headedness or dizziness with exercise.

DIGITALIS	
Crystodigin	Digitoxin
Lanoxin	Digoxin

ALPHA BLOCKERS	
Cardura	Doxazosin
Hytrin	Terazosin
Minipress	Prazosin

COMBINATION ALPHA AND BETA BLOCKERS	
Normodyne	Labetalol
Trandate	Labetalol

ANGIOTENSIN-CONVERTING ENZYME INHIBITORS-ACE INHIBITORS	
Altace	Ramipril
Capoten	Captopril
Capozide	Captopril and Hydrochlorthiazide
Lotensin	Benazepril
Monopril	Fosinopril
Prinivil	Lisinopril
Vasotec	Enalapril
Zestoretic	Lisinopril and Hydrochlorthiazide
Zestril	Lisinopril

Medications that May Affect Your Ability to Exercise

DIURETICS

Bumex	Bumetanide
Edecrin	Ethacrynic acid
Lasix	Furosemide
Aldactazide	Spironolactone and Hydrochlorthiazide
Diucardin	Hydroflumethiazide
Diuril	Chlorthiazide
Dyazide	Triamterene and Hydrochlorthiazide
Enduron	Methyclothiazide
Esidrix	Hydrochlorthiazide
HydroDIURIL	Hydrochlorthiazide
Maxzide	Triamterene and Hydrochlorthiazide
Moduretic	Amiloride and Hydrochlorthiazide
Oretic	Hydrochlorthiazide
Zaroxolyn	Metolazone

Because diuretics increase the loss of sodium and water into the urine, it is possible to become dehydrated if adequate water is not consumed. Exercise under such conditions could be hazardous.

ANTI-ARRHYTHMICS

Cardioquin	Quinidine
Cordarone	Amiodarone
Enkaid	Encainide
Ethmozine	Moricizine
Mexitil	Mexiletine
Norpace	Disopyramide
Procan	Procainamide
Pronestyl	Procainamide
Quinidex	Quinidine
Rythmol	Propafenone
Tambocor	Flecainide
Tonocard	Tocainide

NITROGLYCERINS

Dilatrate	Isosorbide dinitrate
Isordil	Isosorbide dinitrate
Minitran Transdermal	Nitroglycerin patch
NitroBid	Nitroglycerin
Nitrodisc	Nitroglycerin patch
NitroDur	Nitroglycerin patch
Nitrogard	Nitroglycerin
Nitrostat	Nitroglycerin
Peritrate	Pentaerythritol tetranitrate
Sorbitrate	Isosorbide dinitrate
Transderm-Nitro Transdermal	Nitroglycerin patch

Nitroglycerins may cause light-headedness or fainting, particularly if exercise is stopped abruptly.

OTHER ANTIHYPERTENSIVES

Aldomet	Methyldopa
Catapres	Clonidine
Ismelin	Guanethidine
Serapasil	Reserpine
Tenex	Guanfacine
Wytensin	Guanabenz

These may cause blood pressure to drop with exercise. Light-headedness or fainting could result.

PULMONARY DRUGS

Alupent	Metaproterenol
Brethine	Terbutaline
Bronkosol	Isoetharine
Intal	Cromolyn sodium
Provental	Albuterol
Theo-Dur	Aminophylline
Ventolin	Albuterol

These medications may cause the heart rate to abruptly increase.

PERIPHERAL ARTERY DILATORS

Apresoline	Hydralazine
Loniten	Minoxidil
Trental	Pentoxifylline

The blood pressure may drop with these medications, particularly after exercising.

Osteoporosis Support Groups

Support groups are located in many areas across the United States. They offer interested individuals the opportunity to come together to discuss new developments in osteoporosis prevention and treatment and to share personal experiences in coping with the disease. Many support groups have guest speakers and other types of informative programs. Educational materials on osteoporosis, nutrition programs, exercise programs, and physician referrals may also be available through some groups.

ARIZONA
Osteoporosis Awareness Group
University of Arizona
1501 North Campbell, Rm. 6409
Tucson, AZ 85724
Contact: Karen Liebler, R.N.
602-626-2592

CALIFORNIA
Shasta-Area Osteoporosis Awareness Forum
3304-48 Shasta Dam Blvd.
Central Valley, CA 96019
Contact: Helen Fisher
916-275-3800

Davis Senior Center
646 A St.
Davis, CA 95616
Contact: Lisa DeAmicis, Information and
    Referral Coordinator
916-757-5696
Note: This group operates as an educational
organization that meets twice a year.

INDIANA
Osteoporosis Information and Support Group
    of Wayne County
784 Woods Rd.
Richmond, IN 47374
Contact: Margaret Inglis
317-935-5038

KANSAS
Osteoporosis Support Group
University of Kansas
3901 Rainbow Blvd.
Kansas City, KS 66103
Contact: Beth Lucasey, R.N.
913-588-6022

MARYLAND
The Greater Baltimore Osteoporosis Support
    Group
GBMC Conference Center
6565 North Charles St.
Towson, MD 21204
Contact: Treva Zyna
410-356-1101

MASSACHUSETTS
Osteoporosis Support Group of Central
    Massachusetts
M. Elizabeth Fletcher Women's Wellness
    Center (a program of the Fallon
    Healthcare System)
630A Plantation St.
Worcester, MA 01605
508-832-8110
800-891-2300

NEW JERSEY
New Jersey Osteoporosis Society
4316 Finlaw Ave.
Pennsauken, NJ 08109
Contact: Dolores Clark
609-663-1342
800-787-0171

NEW YORK
Living with Osteoporosis
222 Station Plaza N, Ste. 330
Mineola, NY 11501
Contact: Sherri Roth, C.S.W., Program
    Director, RISE
516-663-2920

OREGON
Osteoporosis Support Group of Portland
The Providence Center for Metabolic Bone
    Disorders
Providence Medical Center
4805 NE Glisan St.
Portland, OR 97213
503-215-6586

Medford Osteoporosis Support Group
Rogue Valley Medical Center
Physical Therapy Department
Medford, OR 97504
Contact: Marilyn Duman, 541-664-3266
Call after 12:00 P.M. Pacific time.

PENNSYLVANIA
Nesbit Memorial Hospital
562 Wyoming Ave.
Kingston, PA 18704
Contact: Judi Nowak, R.N., or Margaret
    Petroski
717-283-7222

WASHINGTON
Osteoporosis Awareness Resource
West 2022 Weile Ave.
Spokane, WA 99208
Contact: Lyda C. Johnson, R.N.
509-466-7949

Osteoporosis Support Group of Snohomish
    County
2130 Colby Ave.
Everett, WA 98201
Contact: Betty Morrow
206-252-5242

Recommended Reading

Menopause is an expected event in the life of every woman during which a woman's body undergoes profound changes. Women have many questions about menopause and estrogen replacement that often go unanswered. Two of the recognized authorities in the field of menopause and estrogen replacement have authored superb books, which I recommend to my own patients.

Estrogen—The Facts that Can Change Your Life by Lila Nachtigall, M.D., and Joan Rattner Heilman. New York: Harper & Row, 1986.

Managing Your Menopause by Wulf H. Utian, M.D., Ph.D., and Ruth S. Jacobowitz. New York: Simon & Schuster/Fireside, 1992.

If you would like additional information on osteoporosis, I recommend the following two publications:

Preventing Osteoporosis by Kenneth H. Cooper, M.D., M.P.H., New York: Bantam, 1989.

Stand UP to Osteoporosis by the National Osteoporosis Foundation. Washington, DC: NOF, 1991. This is a 22-page booklet available from the foundation for 40¢ each for the first 200 copies.

Exercise has become a science in and of itself. As women have become more active in competitive sports and as the health benefits of exercise for women have become clear, the need for an authoritative discussion of health and exercise issues unique to women evolved.

Exercise programs that specifically addressed the health concerns of women became necessary. I highly recommend Drs. Mona Shangold and Gabe Mirkin's book and Dr. and Mrs. Cooper's book for all women interested in learning more about exercise programs for women and the effects of exercise on a woman's body.

The Complete Sports Medicine Book for Women by Mona Shangold, M.D., and Gabe Mirkin, M.D. New York: Simon & Schuster/Fireside, 1992.

The New Aerobics for Women by Kenneth Cooper, M.D., M.P.H., and Mildred Cooper. New York: Bantam Books, 1988.

Although osteoarthritis and osteoporosis are two very different diseases, many older women have both. Dr. Neil Gordon's book on exercise and arthritis is recommended reading for anyone who suffers from arthritis.

Arthritis: Your Complete Exercise Guide by Neil F. Gordon, M.D., Ph.D., M.P.H. Champaign, IL: Human Kinetics Publishers, 1993.

Bibliography

Chapter 1 Osteoporosis: The Woman's Epidemic

1. Chrischilles, E.A., et. al. "A Model of Lifetime Osteoporosis Impact." *Archives of Internal Medicine*, (1991) vol. 151, p. 2026–2032.

2. Cummings, S.R., D.M. Black, and S.M. Rubin. "Lifetime Risks of Hip, Colles' or Vertebral Fracture and Coronary Heart Disease Among White Menopausal Women." *Archives of Internal Medicine*, (1989) vol. 149, p. 2445–2448.

3. Phillips, S., et. al. "The Direct Medical Costs of Osteoporosis for American Women Aged 45 and Older, 1986." *Bone*, (1988) vol. 9, p. 271–279.

4. Melton, L.J. "Epidemiology of Age-Related Fractures." *The Osteoporotic Syndrome*. Edited by L.V. Avioli. New York: Wiley Liss, 1993.

5. Obrant, K.J., et. al. "Increasing Age-Adjusted Risk of Fragility Fractures: A Sign of Increasing Osteoporosis in Successive Generations?" *Calcification Tissue International*, (1989) vol. 44, p. 157–167.

6. Melton, L.J., W.M. O'Fallon, and B.L. Riggs. "Secular Trends in the Incidence of Hip Fractures." *Calcification Tissue International*, (1987) vol. 41, p. 57–64.

7. Cooper, C., et. al. "Secular Trends in Postmenopausal Vertebral Fractures." *Calcification Tissue International*, (1992) vol. 51, p. 100–104.

8. Mazess, R.B., et. al. "Spine and Femur Density Using Dual-photon Absorptiometry in U.S. White Women." *Bone and Mineral*, (1987) vol. 2, p. 211–219.

9. Riggs, B.L., et. al. "Differential Changes in Bone Mineral Density of the Appendicular and Axial Skeleton With Aging." *Journal of Clinical Investigation*, (1981) vol. 67, p. 328–335.

10. Mazess, R.B., et. al. "Influence of Age and Body Weight on Spine and Femur Bone Mineral Density in U.S. White Men." *Journal of Bone and Mineral Research*, (1990) vol. 5, p. 645–652.

11. Riggs, B.L., et. al. "Rates of Bone Loss in the Appendicular and Axial Skeletons of Women." *Journal of Clinical Investigation*, (1986) vol. 77, p. 1487–1491.

12. Harris, S. and B. Dawson-Hughes. "Rates of Change in Bone Mineral Density of the Spine, Heel, Femoral Neck, and Radius in Healthy Postmenopausal Women." *Bone and Mineral*, (1992) vol. 17, p. 87–95.

13. Peck, W.A. "Consensus Development Conference: Diagnosis, Prophylaxis, and Treatment of Osteoporosis." *American Journal of Medicine*. (1993) vol. 94, p. 646–650.

14. Kanis, J.A., et al. "The Diagnosis of Osteoporosis." *Journal of Bone and Mineral Research*. (1994) vol. 9, p. 1137–1141.

15. World Health Organization. "Assessment of Fracture Risk and Its Application to Screening for Postmenopausal Osteoporosis." Geneva: WHO, 1994.

Chapter 2 Are You at Risk for Osteoporosis?

1. Cundy, T., et. al. "Bone Density in Women Receiving Medroxyprogesterone Acetate for Contraception." *BMJ*, (1991) vol. 303, p. 13–16.

2. Bianchi, G., et. al. "Effects of Gonadotrophin-releasing Hormone Agonist on Uterine Fibroids and Bone Density." (1989) vol. 11, p. 179–185.

3. Jacobson, J.B. "Effects of Nafarelin on Bone Density." *American Journal of Obstetrics and Gynecology*, (1990) vol. 162, p. 591–592.

4. Riss, B.J., et. al. "Is it possible to Prevent Bone Loss in Young Women Treated With Luteinizing Hormone-releasing Hormone Agonists?" *Journal of Clinical Endocrinology & Metabolism*, (1990) vol. 70, p. 920–924.

5. Pace, J.N., J.L. Miller, and L.J. Rose. "GnRH Agonists: Gonadorelin, Leuprolide, and Nafarelin." *American Journal of Family Practice*, (1991) vol. 44, p. 1777–1782.

6. Mazanec, D.J. and J.M. Grisanti. "Drug-induced Osteoporosis." *Cleveland Clinic Journal of Medicine*, (1989) vol. 56, p. 297–303.

7. Bikle, D.D., et. al. "Bone Disease in Alcohol Abuse." *Annals of Internal Medicine*, (1985) vol. 103, p. 42–48.

8. Seeman, E., et. al. "Reduced Bone Mass in Daughters of Women With Osteoporosis." *New England Journal of Medicine*, (1989) vol. 320, p. 554–558.

9. Matovic, V., et. al. "Factors That Influence Peak Bone Mass Formation: A Study of Calcium Balance and the Inheritance of Bone Mass in Adolescent

Females." *American Journal of Clinical Nutrition*, (1990) vol. 52, p. 878–888.

10. Melton, L.J. and B.L. Riggs. "Clinical Spectrum." *Osteoporosis: Etiology, Diagnosis, and Management*. Edited by B.L. Riggs and L.J. Melton. New York: Raven Press, 1988.

11. Barrett-Connor, E. and T. Holbrook. "Sex Differences in Osteoporosis in Older Adults With Non-insulin Dependent Diabetes Mellitus." *Journal of the American Medical Association*, (1992) vol. 268, p. 3333–3337.

12. Rigotti, N.A., et. al. "Osteoporosis in Women With Anorexia Nervosa." *New England Journal of Medicine*, (1984) vol. 311, p. 1601–1606.

13. Stall, G.M., et. al. "Accelerated Bone Loss in Hypothyroid Patients Overtreated With 1-thyroxine." *Annals of Internal Medicine*, (1990) vol. 113, p. 265–269.

14. Joyce, J.M., et. al. "Osteoporosis in Women With Eating Disorders: Comparison of Physical Parameters, Exercise, and Menstrual Status With SPA and DPA Evaluation. *Journal of Nuclear Medicine*, (1990) vol. 31, p. 325–331.

15. Toh, S.H., B.C. Claunch, and P.H. Brown. "Effect of Hyperthyroidism and its Treatment on Bone Mineral Content." *Archives of Internal Medicine*, (1985) vol. 145, p. 883–886.

16. Spencer, H. and L. Kramer. "Factors Contributing to Osteoporosis." *Journal of Nutrition*, (1986) vol. 116, p. 316–319.

17. Heaney, R.P., et. al. "Calcium Nutrition and Bone Health in the Elderly." *American Journal of Clinical Nutrition*, (1982) vol. 36, p. 986–1013.

18. Greger, J.L. and M. Krystofiak. "Phosphorus Intake of Americans." *Food Technology*, (1982) vol. 36, p. 78–84.

19. Spencer, H., et. al. "Effect of Phosphorus on the Absorption of Calcium and on the Calcium Balance in Man." *Journal of Nutrition*, (1978) vol. 108, p. 447–457.

20. Spencer, H., et. al. "Effect of Small Doses of Phosphorus on the Absorption of Calcium and Phosphorus Metabolism." *American Journal of Clinical Nutrition*, (1982) vol. 36, p. 32–40.

21. Drinkwater, B.L., et. al. "Bone Mineral Content of Amenorrheic Athletes." *New England Journal of Medicine*, (1984) vol. 311, p. 277–281.

22. Abelow, B.J., T.R. Holford, and K.L. Insogna. "Cross-Cultural Association Between Dietary Animal Protein and Hip Fracture: A Hypothesis." *Calcification Tissue International*, (1992) vol. 50, p. 14–18.

Chapter 3 The Importance of Calcium

1. Holbrook, T.L., E. Barrett-Conner, and D.L. Wingard. "Dietary Calcium and Risk of Hip Fracture: 14 Year Prospective Population Study." *Lancet*, (1988) vol. 2, p. 1046–1049.

2. Chapuy, M.C., et. al. "Vitamin D3 and Calcium to Prevent Hip Fractures in Elderly Women." *New England Journal of Medicine*, (1992) vol. 327, p. 1637–1642.

3. Reid, I.R., et. al. "Effect on Calcium Supplementation on Bone Loss in Postmenopausal Women." *New England Journal of Medicine*, (1993) vol. 328, p. 460–464.

4. Dawson-Hughes, B., et. al. "A Controlled Trial of the Effect of Calcium Supplementation on Bone Density in Postmenopausal Women." *New England Journal of Medicine*, (1990) vol. 323, p. 878–883.

5. Shangraw, R.F. "Factors to Consider in the Selection of a Calcium Supplement." *Journal of U.S. Public Health Service*, p. 46–50.

6. Carr, C.J. and R.F. Shangraw. "Nutritional and Pharmaceutical Aspects of Calcium Supplementation." *American Pharmacy*, (1987) vol. ns27, p. 49–57.

7. Heaney, R.P., P.D. Saville, and R.R. Recker. "Calcium Absorption as a Function of Calcium Intake." *Journal of Laboratory and Clinical Medicine*, (1975) vol. 85, p. 881–890.

8. Pak, C.Y.C. and L.V. Avioli. "Factors Affecting Absorbability of Calcium From Calcium Salts and Food." *Calcification Tissue International*, (1988) vol. 43, p. 55–60.

9. Chan, G.M. "Dietary Calcium and Bone Mineral Status of Children and Adolescents." *American Journal of Diseases in Children*, (1991) vol. 145, p. 631–634.

10. Recker, R.R. "Calcium Absorption and Achlorhydria." *New England Journal of Medicine*, (1985) vol. 313, p. 70–73.

11. Heaney, R.P., R.R. Recker, and P.D. Saville. "Calcium Balance and Calcium Requirements in Middle-aged Women." *American Journal of Clinical Nutrition*, (1977) vol. 30, p. 1603–1611.

12. Heaney, R.P., R.R. Recker, and P.D. Saville. "Menopausal Changes in Calcium Balance Performance." *Journal of Laboratory and Clinical Medicine*, (1978) vol. 92, p. 953–963.

13. Lee, C.J., G.S.Lawler, and G.H. Johnson. "Effects of Calcium Supplementation of the Diets with Calcium and Calcium-rich Foods on Bone Density of Elderly Females with Osteoporosis." *American Journal of Clinical Nutrition*, (1981) vol. 34, p. 819–823.

14. Chapuy, M.C., P. Chapuy, and P.J. Meunier. "Calcium and Vitamin D Supplements: Effects on Calcium Metabolism in Elderly People." *American Journal of Clinical Nutrition*, (1987) vol. 46, p. 324–328.

15. Horowitz, M., et. al. "Effect of Calcium Supplementation on Urinary Hydroxyproline in Osteoporotic Postmenopausal Women." *American Journal of Clinical Nutrition*, (1984) vol. 39, p. 857–859.

16. Barrett-Connor, E. "The RDA for Calcium in the Elderly: Too Little, Too Late." *Calcification Tissue International*, (1989) vol. 44, p. 303–307.

17. Nordin, B.E.C. and R.P. Heaney. "Calcium Supplementation of the Diet: Justified by the Present Evidence." *BMJ*, (1990) vol. 300, p. 1056–1060.

18. Johnston, C.C., et. al. "Calcium Supplementation and Increases in Bone Mineral Density in Children." *New England Journal of Medicine*, (1992) vol. 327, p. 82–87.

19. Riis, B., K. Thomsen, and C. Christiansen. "Does Calcium Supplementation Prevent Postmenopausal Bone Loss?" *New England Journal of Medicine*, (1987) vol. 316, p. 173–177.

20. Heaney, R.P., et. al. "Calcium Nutrition and Bone Health in the Elderly." *American Journal of Clinical Nutrition*, (1982) vol. 36, p. 986–1013.

21. Carroll, M.D., S. Abraham., and C.M. Dresser. Dietary Intake Source Data: United States, 1976–1980. Vital and Health Statistics, Series 11, No. 231. National Center for Health Statistics, Public Health Service. Washington, D.C.: U.S. Government Printing Office, March 1983.

22. Recommended Daily Allowances, 10th Edition. Food and Nutrition Board, Commission on Life Sciences, National Research Council. Published by the National Academy Press. 1989.

23. United States Department of Agriculture. Food and Nutrient Intakes of Individual in 1 day in the United States. Spring 1977. Nationwide Food Consumption Survey 1977–1978. USDA, Consumer Nutrition Center, 1980.

24. Matkovic, V., et. al. "Bone Status and Fracture Rates in Two Regions of Yugoslavia." *American Journal of Clinical Nutrition*, (1979) vol. 32, p. 540–549.

25. Abraham, S., et. al. "Dietary Intake Findings, United States 1971–1974." Hyattsville, MD: National Center for Health Statistics, 1977.

26. *Prevention* Magazine's Healthy Women Reader Response Survey. Abacus Custom Research, Inc. Emmanus, PA, January 1993.

27. NIH Consensus Statement. "Optimal Calcium Intake." (1994) vol. 12, p. 1–31.

Chapter 4 Estrogen's Role in Osteoporosis

1. Albright, F., P.H. Smith, and A.M. Richardson. "Postmenopausal Osteoporosis: Its Clinical Features." *JAMA*, (1941) vol. 116, p. 2465–2474.

2. Ettinger, B.F., H.K. Genant, and C.E. Cann. "Long-term Estrogen Replacement Therapy Prevents Bone Loss and Fractures." *Annals of Internal Medicine*, (1985) vol. 102, p. 319–324.

3. Kiel, D.P., et. al. "Hip Fracture and the Use of Estrogens in Postmenopausal Women." *New England Journal of Medicine*, (1987) vol. 317, p. 1169–1174.

4. Christiansen, C., M.S. Christiansen, and I. Transbol. "Bone Mass in Postmenopausal Women After Withdrawal of Oestrogen/ Gestagen Replacement Therapy." *Lancet*, (1981) vol. 1, p. 459–461.

5. Rebar, R.W. and I.B. Spitzer. "The Physiology and Measurement of Hot Flushes." *American Journal of Obstetrics and Gynecology*, (1987) vol. 156, p. 1284–1288.

6. Kaufman, D.W., et. al. "Noncontraceptive Estrogen Use and the Risk of Breast Cancer." *JAMA*, (1984) vol. 252, p. 63–67.

7. Wingo, P.A., et. al. "The Risk of Breast Cancer in Postmenopausal Women Who Have Used Estrogen Replacement Therapy." *JAMA*, (1987) vol. 257, p. 209–215.

8. Dupont, W.D. and D.L. Page. "Menopausal Estrogen Replacement Therapy and Breast Cancer." *Archives of Internal Medicine*, (1991) vol. 151, p. 67–72.

9. Colditz, G.A., et. al. "Prospective Study of Estrogen Replacement Therapy and Risk of Breast Cancer in Postmenopausal Women." *JAMA*, (1990) vol. 262, p. 2648–2653.

10. American College of Physicians Clinical Guidelines. "Guidelines for Counseling Postmenopausal Women

About Preventative Hormone Therapy." *Annals of Internal Medicine*, (1992) vol. 117, p. 1038–1041.

11. Henrich, J.B. "The Postmenopausal Estrogen/ Breast Cancer Controversy." *JAMA*, (1992) vol. 268, p. 1985–1990.

12. Steinberg, K.K., et. al. "A Meta-analysis of the Effect of Estrogen Replacement Therapy on the Risk of Breast Cancer." *JAMA*, (1991) vol. 268, p. 1900–1902.

13. Aitken, J.M. and D.M. Hart. "Osteoporosis After Oophorectomy." *BMJ*, (1973) vol. 3, p. 515–518.

14. Lindsay, R., et. al. "Prevention of Spinal Osteoporosis in Oophorectomized Women." *Lancet*, (1980) p. 1151–1153.

15. Whitehead, M.I., et. al. "Effects of Estrogens and Progestins on the Biochemistry and Morphology of the Postmenopausal Endometrium." *New England Journal of Medicine*, (1981) vol. 305, p. 1599–1605.

16. Gambrell, R.D. "Etrogen-progestogen replacement and Cancer Risk." *Hospital Practice*, (1990) p. 81–100.

17. Mashchak, C.A., et. al. "Comparison of Pharmacodynamic Properties of Various Estrogen Formulations." *American Journal of Obstetrics and Gynecology*, (1982) vol. 144, p. 511–518.

18. Powers, M.S., et. al. "Pharmacokinetics and Pharmacodynamics of Transdermal Dosage Forms of 17-B-Estradiol: Comparison with Conventional Oral Estrogens Used for Hormone Replacement." *American Journal of Obstetrics and Gynecology*, (1982) vol. 152, p. 1099–1106.

19. Harris, S.T., et. al. "The Effects if Estrone (Ogen) on Spinal Bone Density of Postmenopausal Women." *Archives of Internal Medicine*, (1991) vol. 151, p. 1980–1984.

20. Ettinger, B., et. al. "Low-dosage Micronized 17-B-Estradiol Prevents Bone Loss in Postmenopausal Women ." *American Journal of Obstetrics and Gynecology*, (1992) vol. 166, p. 479–488.

21. Lufkin, E.G., et. al. "Treatment of Postmenopausal Osteoporosis with Transdermal Estrogen." *Annals of Internal Medicine*, (1992) vol. 117, p. 1–9.

22. Horsman, A., et. al. "The Effect of Estrogen Dose on Postmenopausal Bone Loss." *New England Journal of Medicine*, (1983) vol. 309, p. 1405–1407.

23. Cann, C.E., et. al. "Decreased Spinal Mineral Content in Amenorrheic Women." *JAMA*, (1984) vol. 251, p. 626–629.

24. Marslew, U., et al. "Bleeding Pattern and Climacteric Symptoms During Different Sequential Combined HRT Regimens in Current Use." *Maturitas.* (1994) vol. 19, p. 225–237.

25. Archer, D.F., J.H. Pickar, and F. Bottiglioni. "Bleeding Patterns in Postmenopausal Women Taking Continuous Combined or Sequential Regimens of Conjugated Estrogen with Medroxyprogesterone Acetate." *Obstetrics and Gynecology.* (1994) vol. 83, p. 686–692.

26. Woodruff, J.D. and J.H. Pickar. "Incidence of Endometrial Hyperplasia in Postmenopausal Women Taking Conjugated Estrogens (Premarin) with Medroxyprogesterone Acetate or Conjugated Estrogens Alone." *American Journal of Obstetrics and Gynecology.* (1994) vol. 170, p. 1213–1223.

Chapter 5 Another Look at Smoking and Caffeine

1. McKinlay, S.M., N.L. Bifano, and J.B. McKinlay. "Smoking and Age at Menopause in Women" *Annals of Internal Medicine*, (1985) vol. 102, p. 350–356.

2. Michnovicz, J.J., et. al. "Increased 2-Hydroxylation of Estradiol as a Possible Mechanism for the Antiestrogenic Effect of Cigarette Smoking." *New England Journal of Medicine*, (1986) vol. 1986, p. 1305–1309.

3. Kiel, D.P., et. al. "Smoking Eliminates the protective Effect of Oral Estrogens on the Risk for Hip Fracture Among Women." *Annals of Internal Medicine*, (1992) vol. 116, p. 716–721.

4. Everson, R.B., et. al. "Effect of Passive Exposure to Smoking on Age at Natural Menopause." *BMJ*, (1986) vol. 293, p. 792.

5. MacMahon, B., et. al. "Cigarette Smoking and Urinary Estrogens." *New England Journal of Medicine*, (1982) vol. 307, p. 1062–1065.

6. Jensen, J., C. Christiansen, and P. Rodbro. "Cigarette Smoking, Serum Estrogens and Bone Loss During Hormone Replacement Therapy Early After Menopause." *New England Journal of Medicine*, (1985) vol. 313, p. 973–975.

7. Pocock, N.A., et. al. "Effects of Tobacco Use on Axial and Appendicular Bone Mineral Density." *Bone*, (1989) vol. 10, p. 329–331.

8. "Caffeine." A Scientific Status Summary of the Institute of Food Technologists' Expert Panel on Food Safety and Nutrition. Institute of Food Technologies, Chicago, Illinois.

9. Heaney, R.P. and R.R. Recker. "Effects on Nitrogen, Phosphorus, and Caffeine on Calcium Balance in

Women." *Journal of Laboratory and Clinical Medicine*, (1982) vol. 99, p. 46–55.

10. Massey, L.K. and K.J. Wise. "The Effect of Dietary Caffeine on Urinary Excretion of Calcium, Magnesium, Phosphorus, Sodium, and Potassium in Healthy Young Females." *Nutrition Research*, (1984) vol. 4, p. 43–50.

11. Massey, L.K. and T.A. Berg. "The Effect of Dietary Caffeine on urinary Excretion Calcium, Magnesium, Phosphorus, Sodium, Potassium, Chloride and Zinc in Healthy Males." *Nutrition Research*, (1985) vol. 5, p. 1281–1284.

12. Barger-Lux, M.J., R.P. Heaney, and M.R. Stegman. "Effects of Moderate Caffeine Intake on the Calcium Economy of Premenopausal Women." *American Journal of Clinical Nutrition*, (1990) vol. 52, p. 722–725.

13. Massey, L.K., D.J. Sherrard, and E.A. Bergman. "Dietary Caffeine Lowers Ultrafiltrable Calcium Levels in Women Consuming Low Dietary Calcium." *Journal of Bone Mineral Research*, (1989) vol. 4, p. S1–249.

Chapter 6 Exercise and Osteoporosis

1. American College of Sports and Medicine. "Guidelines for Exercise testing and Prescription." Philadelphia, PA: Lea and Febiger, 1991.

2. Clarke, D.H. "Training for Strength." *Women and Exercise: Physiology and Sports Medicine*. Ed. by Shangold, M.M. and G, Mirkin. Philadelphia: F.A. Davis Co., 1988.

3. Smith, L. "Bone Concerns." *Women and Exercise: Physiology and Sports Medicine*. Ed. by Shangold, M.M. and G, Mirkin. Philadelphia: F.A. Davis Co., 1988.

4. Shangold, M.M. "Exercise in the Menopausal Woman." *Obstetrics and Gynecology*, (1990) vol. 75, p. 53S–58S.

5. Nilsson, B.E. and N.E. Westlin. "Bone Density in Athletes." Clinical Orthopedic and Related Research, (1971) vol. 77, p. 179–182.

6. Huddleston, A.L., et. al. "Bone Mass in Lifetime Tennis Athletes." *JAMA*, (1980) vol. 244, p. 1107–1109.

7. Brown, A.B., N. McCartney, and D.G. Sale. "Positive Adaptations to Weight-lifting Training in the Elderly." *Journal of Applied Physiology* (1990), vol. 69, p. 1725–1733.

8. Charette, S.L., et. al. "Muscle Hypertrophy Response to Resistance Training in Older Women."

Journal of Applied Physiology, (1991) vol. 70, p. 1912–1916.

9. Colletti, L.A., et. al. "The Effects of Muscles Building Exercise on Bone Mineral Density of the Radius, Spine and Hip in Young Men." *Calcification Tissue International*, (1989) vol. 45, p. 12–14.

10. Sinaki, M. "The Role of Exercising in Preventing Osteoporosis." *Journal of Musculoskeletal Medicine*, (1992) p. 67–83.

11. Simkin, A., J. Ayalon, and I. Leichter. "Increased Trabecular Bone Density Due To Bone-loading Exercises in Postmenopausal Osteoporotic Women." *Calcification Tissue International*, (1987) vol. 40, p. 59–63.

12. Gutin, B. and M.J. Kasper. "Can Vigorous Exercise Play a Role in Osteoporosis Prevention?" *Osteoporosis International*, (1992) vol. 2, p. 55–69.

13. Granhead, H., R. Jonson, and T. Hansson. "The Loads on the Lumbar Spine During Extreme Weight Lifting." *Spine*, (1987) vol. 12, p. 146–149.

14. Aloia, J.F., et. al. "Premenopausal Bone Mass is Related to Physical Activity." *Archives of Internal Medicine*, (1988) vol. 148, p. 121–123.

15. Probart, C.K., et. al. "The Effect of Modern Aerobic Exercise on Physical Fitness Among Women 70 Years or Older." *Maturitus*, (1991) vol. 14, p. 49–56.

16. Dalsky, G.P. "The Role of exercise in the Prevention of Osteoporosis." *Comprehensive Therapy*, (1989) vol. 15, p. 30–37.

17. Dalsky, G.P., et. al. "Weight-bearing Exercise Training and Lumbar Bone Mineral Content in Postmenopausal Women." *Annals of Internal Medicine*, (1988) vol. 1008, p. 824–828.

18. Notelovita, M., et. al. "Estrogen therapy and Variable-resistance Weight Training Increase Bone Mineral in Surgically Menopausal Women." *Journal of Bone Mineral Research*, (1991) vol. 6, p. 583–590.

19. Pruitt, L.A. et. al. "Weight-training Effects of Bone Mineral Density in Early Postmenopausal Women." *Journal of Bone Mineral Research*, (1992) vol. 7, p. 179–185.

20. Sinaki, M. and B.A. Mikkelson. "Postmenopausal Spinal Osteoporosis: Flexion Versus Extension Exercises." *Archives of Physical Medicine and Rehabilitation*, (1984) vol. 65, p. 593–596.

21. Fiatarone, M.A., et. al. "High-intensity Strength Training in Nonagenarians." *JAMA*, (1990) vol. 263, p. 3029–3034.

22. Smith, E.L., et. al. "Deterring Bone Loss by Exercise Intervention in Premenopausal and Postmenopausal Women." *Calcification Tissue International*, (1989) vol. 44, p. 312–321.

23. LeBlanc, A., et. al. "Spinal Bone Mineral After 5 Weeks of Bed Rest." *Calcification Tissue International*, (1987) vol. 41, p. 259–261.

24. Kanders, B., D. Dempster, and R. Lindsay. "Interaction of Calcium Nutrition and Physical Activity on Bone Mass in Young Women." *Journal of Bone Mineral Research*, (1988) vol. 3, p. 145–149.

25. Dawson-Hughes, B., et. al. "Bone Density of the Radius, Spine and Hip in Relation to Percent of Ideal Body Weight in Postmenopausal Women." *Calcification Tissue International*, (1987) vol. 40, p. 310–314.

26. Slemenda, C.W., et. al. "Role of Physical Activity in the Development of Skeletal Mass in Children." *Journal of Bone Mineral Research*, (1991) vol. 6, p. 1227–1233.

Chapter 7 Exercising to Prevent Osteoporosis

1. Wilmore, J.H. "Alterations in Strength, Body Composition, and Anthropometric Measurements Consequent to a 10-Week Weight Training Program." *Medicine and Science in Sports and Exercise*, (1974) vol. 6, p. 133–138.

2. Brown, C.H. and J.H. Wilmore. "The Effects of Maximal Resistance Training on the Strength and Body Composition of Women Athletes." *Medicine and Science In Sports and Exercise*, (1974) vol. 6, p. 174–177.

3. Fleck, S.J. and W.J. Kraemer. *Designing Resistance Exercise Programs*. Campaign, IL: Human Kinetics Books, 1987.

4. Garhammer, J. *Strength Training: Your Ultimate Weight Conditioning Program*. New York: Winner's Circle Books, 1987.

5. Lane, N.E., et. al. "Running, Osteoarthritis, and Bone Density: Initial 2-year Longitudinal Study." *American Journal of Medicine*, (1990) vol. 88, p. 452–459.

Chapter 8 Exercise for the Women with Osteoporosis

1. Sinaki, M. "Exercise and Physical Therapy." *Osteoporosis: Etiology, Diagnosis and Management*. Ed. Riggs, B.L. and L.J. Melton. New York: Raven Press, 1988.

2. Sinaki, M. and B.A. Mikkelsen. "Postmenopausal Spinal Osteoporosis: Flexion Versus Extension Exercises." *Archives of Physical Medicine and Rehabilitation*, (1984) vol. 65, p. 593–596.

3. Sinaki, M. "The Role of Exercise in Preventing Osteoporosis." *Journal of Musculoskeletal Medicine*, (1992) p. 67–83.

Chapter 9 Vitamin D

1. Dawson-Hughes, B., et. al. "Effect of Vitamin D Supplementation on Wintertime and Overall Bone Loss in Healthy Postmenopausal Women." *Annals of Internal Medicine*, (1991) vol. 115, p. 505–512.

2. Chapuy, M.C., et. al. "Vitamin D3 and Calcium to Prevent Hip Fractures in Elderly Women." *New England Journal of Medicine*, (1992) vol. 327, p. 1637–1642.

3. Slovik, D.M., et. al. "Deficient Production of 1, 25 Dihydroxyvitamin D in Elderly Osteoporotic Patients." *New England Journal of Medicine*, (1981) vol. 305, p. 372–374.

4. Tilyard, J. "Low-dose Calcitriol Versus Calcium in Established Postmenopausal Osteoporosis." *Metabolism*, (1990) vol. 39, p. S50–52.

5. Gallagher, J.C. and B.L. Riggs. "Action of 1, 25 Dihydroxyvitamin D3 on Calcium Balance and Bone Turnover and its Effect on Vertebral Fracture Rate." *Metabolism*, (1990) vol. 39, p. S30–34.

6. Aloia, J. "The Role of Calcitriol in the Treatment of Postmenopausal Osteoporosis." *Metabolism*, (1990) vol. 39, p. S35–38.

7. Riggs, B.L. and K.I. Nelson. "Effect of Long-term Treatment with Calcitriol on Calcium Absorption and Mineral Metabolism in Postmenopausal Osteoporosis." *Journal of Clinical Endocrinology and Metabolism*, (1985) vol. 61, p. 457–461.

Chapter 10 Other Vitamins, Other Minerals

1. Carmel, R., et. al. "Cobalamin and Osteoblast-specific Proteins." *New England Journal of Medicine*, (1988) vol. 319, p. 70–75.

2. Rico, H. "Minerals and Osteoporosis." *Osteoporosis International*, (1991) vol. 2, p. 20–25.

3. Beattie, J.H. and A. Avenell. "Trace Element Nutrition and Bone Metabolism." *Nutrition Research Reviews*, (1992) vol. 5, p. 167–188.

4. "Nutrition Management." *The Johns Hopkins Handbook*. Ed. by Walser, M., et. al. Philadelphia: W.B. Saunders Co., 1984.

5. "Bowes and Church's Food Values of Portions Commonly Used." Ed. by Pennington, J.A.T. and H.N. Church. Philadelphia: J.B. Lippincott Co., 1985.

6. Heaney, R.P. "Nutritional factors in Bone Health." *Osteoporosis, Etiology, Diagnosis and Management.* Ed. by Riggs, B.L. and L.J. Melton. New York: Raven Press, 1988.

7. Chandra, R.K. "Effect of Vitamin and Trace-element Supplementation on Immune Responses and Infection in Elderly Subjects." *Lancet*, (1992) vol. 340, p. 1124–1127.

Chapter 11 Preventing Falls

1. Tinetti, M.E., M. Speechley, and S.F. Ginger. "Risk Factors for Falls Among Elderly Persons Living in the Community." *New England Journal of Medicine*, (1988) vol. 319, p. 1701–1706.

2. Rubenstein, L.Z., et. al. "The Value of Assessing Falls in Elderly Population." *Annals of Internal Medicine*, (1990) vol. 113, p. 308–316.

3. Hindmarsh, J.J. and E.H. Estes. "Falls in Older Persons." *Archives of Internal Medicine*, (1989) vol. 149, p. 2217–2222.

4. Tinetti, M.E., W. Lin, and E.B. Claus. "Predictors and Prognosis of Inability to Get Up After Falls Among Elderly Persons." *JAMA*, (1993) vol. 269, p. 65–70.

5. Tinetti, M.E. and M. Speechley. "Prevention of Falls Among the Elderly." *New England Journal of Medicine*, (1989) vol. 320, p. 1055–1059.

6. Peck, W.A. "Falls and Hip Fracture in the Elderly." *Hospital Practice*, (1986) p. 72A–72K.

7. Ensrud, K.E., et. al. "Postural hypotension and Postural Dizziness in Elderly Women." *Archives of Internal Medicine*, (1992) vol. 152, p. 1057–1064.

8. Felson, D.T. "Prevention of Hip Fractures." *Hospital Practice*, (1988) p. 23–38.

9. Ray, W.A., et. al. "Psychotropic Drug Use and the Risk of Hip Fracture." *New England Journal of Medicine*, (1987) vol. 316, p. 363–369.

Chapter 12 Bone Density Testing

1. Johnston, C.C., C.W. Slemenda and L.J. Melton. "Clinical use of Bone Densitometry." *New England Journal of Medicine*, (1991) vol. 324, p. 1105–1109.

2 . Rubin, S.M. and S.R. Cummings. "Results of Bone Densitometry Affect Women's Decisions About Taking Measures to Prevent Fractures." *Annals of Internal Medicine*, (1992) vol. 116, p. 990–995.

3. Cummings, S.R., et. al. "Appendicular Bone Density and Age Predict Hip Fracture in Women." *JAMA*, (1990) vol. 263, p. 665–707.

4. Genant, H.K., et. al. "Quantitative Computer Tomograph of Vertebral Spongiosa: A Sensitive Method for Detecting Early Bone Loss After Oophorectomy." *Annals of Internal Medicine*, (1982) vol. 97, p. 699–705.

5. Ross, P.D., et. al. "Definition of a Spine Fracture Threshold Based Upon Prospective Fracture Risk." *Bone*, (1987) vol. 271–278.

6. Pouilles, J.M., et. al. "Risk Factors of Vertebral Osteoporosis. Results of a Study of 2279 Women Referred to a Menopause Clinic." *Rev. Rhum. Mal. Osteoarticulaires*, (1991) vol. 58, p. 169–177.

7. Hui, S.L., C.W. Slemenda and C.C. Johnston. "Baseline Measurement of Bone Mass Predicts Fracture in White Women." *Annals of Internal Medicine*, (1989) vol. 111, p. 355–361.

8. Melton, L.J., et. al. "Long-term Fracture Risk Prediction with Bone Mineral Measurements Made at Various Sites." Abstract presented at the American Society for Bone and Mineral Research meeting, August 25, 1991.

9. Hui, S.L., C.W. Slemenda and C.C. Johnston. "Age and Bone Mass as Predictors of Fracture in a Prospective Study." *Journal of Clinical Investigation*, (1988) vol. 81, p. 1804–1809.

10. Mazess, R.B. and H.S. Barden. "Measurement of Bone by Dual-photon Absorptiometry (dpa) and Dual-energy Xray Absorptiometry (dexa)." *Annales Chirugiae et Gynaecologiae*, (1988) vol. 77, p. 197–203.

11. Health and Public Policy Committee, American College of Physicians. "Radiologic Methods to Evaluate Bone Mineral Content." *Annals of Internal Medicine*, (1984) vol. 100, p. 908–911.

12. Scientific Advisory Board of National Osteoporosis Foundation." "Clinical Indications for Bone Mass Measurements." *Journal of Bone and Mineral Research*, (1989) vol. 4 (S2), p. 1–28.

13. Wasnich, R.D., et. al. "A Comparison of Single and Multi-site BMC Measurements for Assessment of Spine Fracture Probability." *Journal of Nuclear Medicine*, (1989) vol. 30, p. 1166–1171.

14. Wasnich, R.D., et. al. "Prediction of Post-menopausal Fracture Risk with Use of Bone Mineral Measurements." *American Journal of Obstetrics and Gynecology*, (1985) vol. 153, p. 745–751.

15. Kalender, W.A. "Effective Dose Values in Bone Mineral Measurements by Photon Absorptiometry and Computed Tomograph." *Osteoporosis International,* (1992) vol. 2, p. 82–87.

16. Clark, A.P. and J.A. Schuttinga. "Targeted Estrogen/Progestogen Replacement Therapy for osteoporosis: Calculation of Health Care Cost Savings." *Osteoporosis International,* (1992) vol. 2, p. 195–200.

Chapter 13 Salmon Calcitonin in the Treatment of Osteoporosis

1. Rico, H., et. al. "Salmon Calcitonin Reduces Vertebral Fracture Rate in Postmenopausal Crush Fracture Syndrome." *Bone and Mineral,* (1992) vol. 16, p. 113–128.

2. Mazzuoli, G.F., et. al. "Effects of Salmon Calcitonin on the Bone Loss Induced by Ovariectomy." *Calcification Tissue International,* (1990) vol. 47, p. 209–214.

3. Mazzuoli, G.F., et. al. "Effects of Salmon Calcitonin in Postmenopausal Osteoporosis: A Controlled Double-blind Clinical Study." *Calcification Tissue International,* (1986) vol. 38, p. 3–8.

4. Reginster, J.Y., et. al. "One Year Controlled Randomized Trial of Prevention of Early Postmenopausal Bone Loss by Intranasal Calcitonin." *Lancet,* (1987) vol. 2, p. 1481–1483.

5. Civitelli, R., et. al. "Bone Turnover in Postmenopausal Osteoporosis: Effect of Calcitonin Treatment." *Journal of Clinical Investigation,* (1988) vol. 82, p. 1268–1274.

6. Reginster, J.Y. "Management of High Turnover Osteoporosis with Calcitonin." *Bone,* (1992) vol. 13, p. S37–S40.

7. MacIntyre, I., et. al. "Calcitonin for Prevention of Postmenopausal Bone Loss." *Lancet,* (1988) vol. 1, p. 900–901.

8. McDermott, M.T. and G.S. Kidd. "The Role of Calcitonin in the development and treatment of Osteoporosis." Endocrine Reviews, (1987) vol. 8, p. 377–390.

9. Levernieux, J., D. Julien and F. Caulin. "A Double-blind Study on the Effect of Calcitonin on Pain and Acute Resorption Related to Recent Osteoporotic Crush Fractures." *Calcitonin 1984: Selected Short Communications, International Symposium Calcitonin 1984 Milan.* Ed. by Doepfner, W. Amsterdam: Excerpta Medica, 1986.

10. Gennari, C. "Comparative Effects on Bone Mineral Content of Calcium Plus Salmon Calcitonin Given in Two Different Regimens in Postmenopausal Osteoporosis." *Current Therapeutics and Research,* (1985) vol. 28, p. 455–464.

11. Adami, S., et al. "Treatment of Postmenopausal Osteoporosis with Continuous Daily Oral Alendronate in Comparison with Either Placebo or Intranasal Salmon Calcitonin." *Osteoporosis International.* (1993) supp. 3, S21–7.

12. Gruber, H.E., et al. "Long-term Calcitonin Therapy in Postmenopausal Osteoporosis." *Metabolism.* (1984) vol. 33, p. 295–303.

13. Wallach, S. "Calcitonin Treatment in Osteoporosis." *Drug Therapy.* (April 1993): 61–74.

14. Lyritis, G.P., etal. "Analgesic Effect of Salmon Calcitonin in Osteoporotic Vertebral Fractures: A Double-Blind Placebo-Controlled Clinical Study." *Calcified Tissue International.* (1991) vol. 49, p. 369–372.

15. Ringe, J.D. and D. Welzel. "Salmon Calcitonin in the Therapy of Corticoid-Induced Osteoporosis." *European Journal of Clinical Pharmacology.* (1987) vol. 33, p. 35–39.

16. Montemurro, L., et al. "Prevention of Corticosteroid-Induced Osteoporosis with Salmon Calcitonin in Sarcoid Patients." *Calcified Tissue International.* (1991) vol. 49, p. 71–76.

17. Overgaard, K., et al. "Effect of Salcatonin Given Intranasally on Bone Mass and Fracture Rates in Established Osteoporosis: A Dose-Response Study." *BMJ.* (1992) vol. 305, p. 556–561.

18. Product Monograph: Miacalcin Nasal Spray. East Hanover, NJ: Sandoz Pharmaceuticals, 1995.

Chapter 14

1. Watts, N.B., et al. "Intermittent Cyclical Etidronate Treatment of Postmenopausal Osteoporosis." *New England Journal of Medicine.* (1990) vol. 323, p. 73–79.

2. Storm, T., et al. "Effect of Intermittent Cyclical Etidronate Therapy of Bone Mass and Fracture Rate in Women with Postmenopausal Osteoporosis." *New England Journal of Medicine.* (1990) vol. 322, p. 1265–1271.

3. Adami, S., et al. "Treatment of Postmenopausal Osteoporosis with Continuous Daily Oral Alendronate in Comparison with Either Placebo or Intranasal Salmon Calcitonin." *Osteoporosis International.* (1993) supp. 3: S21–7.

4. Harris, S.T., et al. "Four-Year Study of Intermittent Cyclical Etidronate Treatment of Postmenopausal Osteoporosis: Three Years of Blinded Therapy Followed by One Year of Open Therapy." *American Journal of Medicine.* (1993) vol. 95, p. 557–567.

5. Marcus, R. "Cyclic Etidronate: Has the Rose Lost Its Bloom?" *American Journal of Medicine.* (1993) vol. 95, p. 555–556.

6. Papapoulos, S.E., et al. "The Use of Bisphosphonates in the Treatment of Osteoporosis." *Bone.* (1992) vol. 13: S41–9.

7. Licata, A.A. "From Bathtub Ring to Osteoporosis: A Clinical Review of the Bisphosphonates." *Cleveland Clinic Journal of Medicine.* (1993) vol. 60, p. 284–290.

8. Gertz, B.J. "Monitoring Bone Resorption in Early Postmenopausal Women by an Immunoassay for Cross-linked Collagen Peptides in Urine." *Journal of Bone and Mineral Research.* (1994) vol. 9, p. 135–142.

9. Reid, I.R. "Treatment of Osteoporosis in Postmenopausal Women with Oral Alendronate." XII International Conference on Calcium Regulating Hormones, 1995. Melbourne, Australia.

10. Reid, I.R., et al. "Two-Year Follow-Up of Bisphosphonate (APD) Treatment in Steroid Osteoporosis." *Lancet.* (1988) vol. 2, p. 1144.

11. Adachi, J., et al. "Intermittent Cyclical Etidronate Therapy Prevents Corticosteroid-Induced Bone Loss." *Arthritis and Rheumatism.* (1993) vol. 36, S51.

12. Liberman, U.A., et al. "Effect of Oral Alendronate on Bone Mineral Density and the Incidence of Fractures in Postmenopausal Women." *New England Journal of Medicine.* (1995) vol. 333, p. 1437–1443.

13. McClung, M., et al. "Risedronate Treatment of Postmenopausal Women with Low Bone Mass: Preliminary Data." (Abstract.) World Congress on Osteoporosis, May 1996. Amsterdam.

Chapter 15 Future Therapies for Osteoporosis

Thiazides

1. LaCroix, A.Z., et. al. "Thiazide Diuretic Agents and the Incidence of Hip Fracture." *New England Journal of Medicine,* (1990) vol. 322, p. 286–290.

2. Wasnich, R.D., et. al. "Thiazide Effect on the Mineral Content of Bone." *New England Journal of Medicine,* (1983) vol. 309, p. 344–347.

3. Felson, D.T., et. al. "Thiazide Diuretics and the Risk of Hip Fracture." *JAMA,* (1991) vol. 265, p. 370–373.

4. Heidrich, F.E., A. Stergachis and K.M. Gross. "Diuretic Drug Use and the Risk of Hip Fracture." *Annals of Internal Medicine,* (1991) vol. 115, p. 1–6.

5. Cauey, J.A., et. al. "Effects of Thiazide Diuretic Therapy on Bone Mass, Fractures and Falls." *Annals of Internal Medicine,* (1993) vol. 118, p. 666–673.

6. Genazzani, A.R., et al. "Org OD 14 and the Endometrium." *Maturitas.* (1991) vol. 13, p. 243-251.

7. Lindsay, R., et al. "Prospective Double-Blind Trial of Synthetic Steroid (Org OD 14) for Preventing Postmenopausal Osteoporosis." *British Medical Journal.* (1980) vol. 1, p. 1207–1209.

8. Rymer, J., et al. "Effect of Tibolone on Postmenopausal Bone Loss." *Osteoporosis International.* (1994) vol. 4, p. 314–319.

9. Rymer, J., et al. "A Study of the Effect of Tibolone on the Vagina in Postmenopausal Women." *Maturitas.* (1994) vol. 18, p. 127–133.

10. Hardiman, P., et al. "Cardiovascular effects of Org OD 14: A New Steroidal Therapy for Climacteric Symptoms." *Maturitas.* (1991) vol. 13, p. 235–242.

Didronel

11. Watts, N.B., et. al. "Intermittent Cyclical Etidronate Treatment of Postmenopausal Osteoporosis." *New England Journal of Medicine,* (1990) vol. 323, p. 73–79.

12. Storm, T, et. al. "Effect of Intermittent Cyclical Etidronate Therapy of Bone Mass and Fracture Rate in Women with Postmenopausal Osteoporosis." *New England Journal of Medicine,* (1990) vol. 322, p. 1265–1271.

13. Jackson, R.D., et. al. "Cyclical Etidronate Treatment of Postmenopausal Osteoporosis: 4 Year Experience." Eleventh International Conference on Calcium Regulating Hormones. Florence, Italy, April 24–29, 1992.

14. Storm, T., et. al. "Five Years of Intermittent Cyclical Etidronate Therapy Increases Bone Mass and Reduces Vertebral Fracture Rate in Postmenopausal Women." Eleventh International Conference on Calcium Regulating Hormones. Florence, Italy, April 24–29, 1992.

15. Papapoulos, S.E.,et. al. "The Use of Biophosphonates in the Treatment of Osteoporosis." *Bone,* (1992) vol. 13, p. S41–S49.

16. Smith, M.L., et. al. "Effect of Etidronate Disodium on Bone Turnover Following Surgical Menopause." *Calcification Tissue International,* (1989) vol. 44, p. 74–79.

Flavanoids

17. Brandi, M.L. "Flavanoids: Biochemical Effects and Therapeutic Applications." *Bone and Mineral,* (1992) vol. 19, p. S3–S14.

18. Passeri, M., et. al. "Effect of Ipriflavone on Bone Mass in Elderly Osteoporotic Women." *Bone and Mineral,* (1992) vol. 19, S57–S62.

Anrogens

19. Gennari, C., et. al. "Effects of Nandrolone Decanoate Therapy on Bone Mass and Calcium Metabolism in Women with Established Post-menopausal Osteoporosis: A Double-blind Placebo-controlled Study." *Maturitas,* (1989) vol. 11, p. 187–197.

20. Need, A.G., et. al. "Effects of Nandrolone Decanoate on Forearm Mineral Density and Calcium Metabolism in Osteoporotic Postmenopausal Women." *Calcification Tissue International,* (1987) vol. 41, p. 7–10.

Nasal Spray Calcitonin

21. Thamsborg, G., et. al. "Effect of Different Doses of Nasal Salmon Calcitonin on Bone Mass." *Calcitonin Tissue International,* (1991) vol. 48, p. 302–307.

Sodium Fluorides

22. Heaney, R.P., et. al. "Fluoride Therapy for the Vertebral Crush Fracture Syndrome: A Status Report." *Annals of Internal Medicine,* (1989) vol. 111, p. 678–680.

23. Riggs, B.L., et. al. "Effect of the Fluoride/Calcium Regimen on Vertebral Fracture Occurrence in Postmenopausal Osteoporosis." *New England Journal of Medicine,* (1982) vol. 306, p. 446–450.

24. O'Duffey, J.D., et. al. "Mechanism of Acute Lower Extremity Pain Syndrome in Fluoride-treated Osteoporotic Patients." *American Journal of Medicine,* (1986) vol. 80, p. 561–566.

25. Hedlund, L.R. and J.C. Gallagher. "Increased Incidence of Hip Fracture in Osteoporotic Women Treated with Sodium Fluoride." *Journal of Bone and Mineral Research,* (1989) vol. 4, p. 223–225.

26. Pak, C.Y.C., et. al. "Safe and effective Treatment of Osteoporosis with Intermittent Slow Release Sodium Fluoride: Augmentation of Vertebral Bone Mass and Inhibition of Fractures." *Journal of Clinical Endocrinology and Metabolism,* (1989) vol. 68, p. 150–159.

27. Riggs, B.L., et. al. "Effect of Fluoride Treatment on the Fracture rate in Postmenopausal Women with Osteoporosis." *New England Journal of Medicine,* (1990) vol. 322, p. 802–809.

28. Riggs, B.L., et al. "Clinical Trial of Fluoride Therapy in Postmenopausal Osteoporotic Women: Extended Observations and Additional Analysis." *Journal of Bone and Mineral Research.* (1994) vol. 9, p. 265–75.

29. Pak, C.Y.C., et al. "Treatment of Postmenopausal Osteoporosis with Slow-Release Sodium Fluoride: Final Update of a Randomized Controlled Trial." *Annals of Internal Medicine.* (1995) vol. 123, p. 401–408.

30. Pak, C.Y.C., et al. "Controlled Comparison of a Nonrandomized Trial with Slow-Release Sodium Fluoride with a Randomized Controlled Trial in Postmenopausal Osteoporosis." *Journal of Bone and Mineral Research.* (1996) vol. 11, p. 160–168.

31. Pak, C.Y.C., et al. "Perspective: Slow-Release Sodium Fluoride in Osteoporosis." *Journal of Bone and Mineral Research.* (1996) vol. 11, p. 561–564.

Calcitriol

32. Riggs, B.L. and K.I. Newman. "Effect of Long-term Treatment with Calcitriol on Calcium Absorption and Mineral Metabolism in Postmenopausal Osteoporosis." *Journal of Clinical Endocrinology and Metabolism,* (1985) vol. 61, p. 457–461.

33. Gallagher, J.C. and D. Goldgar. "Treatment of Postmenopausal Osteoporosis with High Doses of Synthetic Calcitriol." *Annals of Internal Medicine,* (1990) vol. 113, p. 649–655.

34. Slovik, D.M., et. al. "Deficient Production of 1,25 Dihydroxyvitamin D in Elderly Osteoporotic Patients." *New England Journal Of Medicine,* (1981) vol. 305, p. 372–374.

35. Tilyard, M. "Low-dose Calcitriol Versus Calcium in Established Postmenopausal Osteoporosis." *Metabolism,* (1990) vol. 39, p. S50–S52.

36. Aloia, J.F. "Role of Calcitriol in the Treatment of Postmenopausal Osteoporosis." *Metabolism*, (1990) vol. 39, p. S35–S38.

37. Caniggia, A., et. al. "Long-term Treatment with Calcitriol in Postmenopausal Osteoporosis." *Metabolism*, (1990) vol. 39, p. S43–S49.

38. Francis, R.M. and M. Peacock. "Local Action of Oral 1,25 Dihydroxycholecalciferol on Calcium Absorption in Osteoporosis." *American Journal of Clinical Nutrition*, (1987) vol. 46, p. 315–318.

Chapter 16 Osteoporosis in Men

1. Jackson, J.A. and M. Kleerekoper. "Osteoporosis in Men: Diagnosis, Pathophysiology, and prevention." *Medicine*, (1990) vol. 69, p. 137–152.

2. Seeman, E., et. al. "Risk Factors for Spinal Osteoporosis in Men." *American Journal of Medicine*, (1983) vol. 75, p. 977–983.

3. Riggs, B.L., et. al. "Differential Changes in Bone Mineral Density of the Appendicular and Axial Skeleton with Aging." *Journal of Clinical Investigation*, (1981) vol. 67, p. 328–335.

4. Kelly, P.J., et. al. "Dietary Calcium, Sex Hormones, and Bone Mineral Density in Men." *British Medical Journal*, (1990) vol. 300, p. 1361–1364.

5. Drinka, P.J., S.F. Bauwens and A.A. DeSmet. "Atraumatic Vertebral Deformities in Elderly Males." *Calcification Tissue International*, (1987) vol. 41, p. 299–302.

6. Slemenda, C.W., J.C. Christian and T. Reed. "Long-term Bone Loss in Men: Effects of Genetic and Environmental Factors." *Annals of Internal Medicine*, (1992) vol. 117, p. 286–291.

Additional Resources

General Information

National Osteoporosis Foundation
1150 17th Street, N.W., Ste. 500
Washington, DC 20036-4603
202-223-2226
800-223-9994

North American Menopause Society
c/o Cleveland Menopause Clinic
29001 Cedar Rd., No. 600
Cleveland, OH 44124

The Arthritis Foundation
National Office
1314 Spring St., N.W.
Atlanta, GA 30309
404-872-7100

National Arthritis and Musculoskeletal and
    Skin Diseases Information Clearinghouse
Box AMS
Bethesda, MD 20982
301-496-4000

National Dairy Board
National Dairy Council
10255 W. Higgins Rd., Ste. 900
Rosemont, IL 60018
847-803-2000

American College of Obstetricians and
    Gynecologists
409 12th St., S.W.
Washington, DC 20024
202-638-5577

American Academy of Orthopedic Surgeons
6300 N. River Rd.
Rosemont, IL 60018
847-823-7186

Health and Medical Research Foundation
4900 Broadway
San Antonio, TX 78209
210-824-4200

For locations of bone-density testing facilities in your area call:

LUNAR Corp.
313 W. Beltline Hwy.
Madison, WI 53713
800-445-8627

Hologic
590 Lincoln St.
Waltham, MA 02154
800-343-XRAY
(Ask for Nancy Salt)

Norland Corp.
Customer Service Department
W6340 Hackbarth Rd.
Fort Atkinson, WI 53538
800-444-8456

Optimal Health Products & Services
4900 Broadway
San Antonio, TX 78209
210-824-2099

Medical Equipment Supply

North Coast Medical, Inc.
187 Stauffer Blvd.
San Jose, CA 95125-1042
800-821-9319

Glossary

A

Abdominal hysterectomy—See hysterectomy. The surgical removal of the uterus or womb through an incision in the abdomen.

Absorptiometry—See densitometry. A type of medical test to measure the bone density.

Aerobic exercise—Continuous, rhythmic exercise that uses the large muscles of the body for greater than 3 minutes using oxygen for muscle fuel.

Aerobics—A popular term for aerobic exercise. Many people attribute the origin of this term to Dr. Kenneth Cooper.

Alendronate—The chemical name for the new bisphosphonate drug Fosamax, which is manufactured by Merck & Company. This drug was approved by the FDA for the treatment of osteoporosis in 1995.

Amenorrhea—The lack of menstrual periods.

Androgens—A group of hormones related to the male sex hormone testosterone.

Anaerobic—Literally means without oxygen.

Anaerobic exercise—Exercise that requires quick, short bursts of activity in which the muscles use fuel other than oxygen.

Anorexia nervosa—An eating disorder in which individuals starve themselves to death because they believe they are fat. The group most affected by this disorder is primarily made up of young women. This disorder may cause osteoporosis.

Arteriosclerosis—Hardening of the arteries. See atherosclerosis.

Arthritis—An inflammation of the joints that may cause pain, swelling, and redness of the joint. The joint may be destroyed in severe cases.

Atherosclerosis—See arteriosclerosis.

Atrophic—This term describes a condition of deterioration.

Atrophic vaginitis—A thinning and general poor quality of the vaginal tissue, caused by estrogen deficiency and which leads to irritation, infections, and painful intercourse.

B

Bilateral salpingo-oophorectomy—The surgical removal of both ovaries and both fallopian tubes.

Birth control pills—See oral contraceptives.

Bisphosphonates—A group of drugs that are similar to a naturally occurring compound called pyrophosphate that is found in bone. Fosamax belongs to this group of drugs.

Bone densitometry—Medical testing to measure the bone density or strength.

Bone density—The amount of mineral in any given volume of bone. For example, a bone containing 20 g of mineral that is 16.7 square centimeters in size has a bone density of 1.2 g/cm^2.

Bone mass—The amount of mineral in a bone. Although this is different from the bone density, the terms are often used interchangeably.

C

Caffeine—A chemical stimulant commonly found in coffee, tea, and cola-based soft drinks. Excessive caffeine consumption is considered a risk factor for osteoporosis because it increases the urinary loss of calcium.

Calciferol—Another name for vitamin D_2, which comes from plants.

Calcifediol—Another name for 25 hydroxy-vitamin D_3, a form of vitamin D produced in the liver. See Calderol.

Calcimar—Rhone-Poulenc Rorer Pharmaceuticals' prescription form of salmon calcitonin, which is approved by the FDA for the treatment of osteoporosis.

Calcitonin—A hormone produced in the thyroid gland that inhibits bone loss. Synthetic calcitonin from salmon is used in the treatment of osteoporosis.

Calcitriol—Another name for 1,25 dihydroxy-vitamin D, a form of vitamin D produced in the kidneys. See Rocaltrol.

Calcium—The most important mineral found in bone.

Calcium carbonate—A naturally occurring form of calcium, which is commonly used in calcium supplements. Oyster shell calcium is a form of calcium carbonate.

Calcium citrate—A man-made form of calcium used in calcium supplements.

Calcium phosphate—A type of calcium that occurs naturally in milk. It is also used in calcium supplements.

Calderol—The brand name for a prescription form of 25 hydroxy-vitamin D$_3$, which is manufactured by Organon Pharmaceuticals.

Cervical spine—The seven bones or vertebrae in the neck.

Change of life—A phrase that refers to menopause.

Cholesterol—A fatty substance found in the body from which some hormones are made. It has also been implicated in causing arteriosclerosis.

Cholelithiasis—The medical term for gallstones.

Ciba Pharmaceuticals—The pharmaceutical company that makes Estraderm™ (estradiol transdermal system), an estrogen patch that has been approved by the FDA for the prevention of osteoporosis.

Climacteric—The symptoms and signs of estrogen deficiency that occur around the time of menopause.

Climacteric syndrome—Refers to a woman who is experiencing symptoms of estrogen deficiency, such as hot flashes.

Colles' fracture—A type of wrist fracture commonly seen in osteoporosis.

Compression fracture—A fracture of a vertebra or bone in the spine in which the bone collapses rather than breaking in two.

Computerized axial tomography—A three-dimensional X-ray technique that can be used to measure the bone density. Often called a CT or CAT scan.

Conjugated equine estrogen—A form of estrogen replacement for postmenopausal women that is derived from the urine of pregnant mares. Premarin is a form of conjugated equine estrogen.

Contraception—The prevention of pregnancy.

Contraceptive—A pill or device that can be used to prevent pregnancy.

Corpus luteum—The structure in the ovary that produces estrogen and progesterone after ovulation.

Corticosteroids—Refers to substances produced in the adrenal gland or to certain types of medications that are similar to cortisone.

Crush fracture—The total collapse of a vertebra or bone in the spine.

Cyclic treatment regimen—The intermittent but regular administration of a medication to treat disease.

D

Densitometry—See absorptiometry. A type of medical test used to measure the bone mass or density.

Didronel—The brand name of etidronate manufactured by Proctor & Gamble Pharmaceuticals. It is used in the treatment of Paget's disease and is being evaluated in research studies as a treatment for osteoporosis.

Dorsal spine—An older term for the thoracic spine, the region of the spine between the base of the neck and the waist. It consists of 12 individual bones or vertebra.

Dual energy X-ray absorptiometry—A type of bone-density testing that uses X ray to measure the bone density. Many experts believe this technique is the state of the art. Often abbreviated as DEXA or DXA.

Dual photon absorptiometry—A type of bone-density testing that uses a radioactive isotope to measure the bone density. It was the forerunner for dual energy X-ray absorptiometry. Often abbreviated DPA.

E

Endometrial hyperplasia—A precancerous condition of the endometrium or lining of the uterus.

Endometriosis—A disease in which endometrial tissue is found in other areas besides the interior of the uterus. This abnormal tissue can cause bleeding and pain.

Endometrium—The lining of the uterus or womb.

Endorphins—Chemical substances produced in the brain that may act as the body's own natural pain killers.

ERT—The abbreviation for estrogen replacement therapy.

Estrace—An oral estrogen tablet manufactured by Bristol-Myers Squibb that has been approved by the FDA for the prevention of osteoporosis. This is an oral tablet containing 17-beta estradiol.

Estraderm™ (estradiol transdermal system)—An estrogen patch manufactured by Ciba that has been FDA approved for the prevention of osteoporosis. This patch contains estradiol.

Estradiol—The major type of estrogen that is produced by the ovaries.

Estradiol, 17-Beta—A more specific name for estradiol. This is the type of estrogen found in the oral tablet Estrace and the estrogen patch Estraderm™.

Estriol—A third type of estrogen found in women. It has very weak activity in the body.

Estrogen—The female sex hormone produced by the ovaries. There are several types of

estrogen such as estradiol, estrone, and estriol.

Estrone—The second most important type of estrogen found in women.

Estrone sulfate—The form of estrogen found in Ogen, an oral estrogen tablet manufactured by Abbott Laboratories that has been FDA approved for the prevention of osteoporosis.

Etidronate—See Didronel or diphosphonates. A drug used in the treatment of Paget's disease that is currently being evaluated as a possible treatment for osteoporosis.

Extension exercises—This refers to exercises in which the movement of a joint causes the limbs above and below it to move away from one another. In the case of the spine, the spine is arched backward during this type of exercise. This type of spine exercise is considered safe for women with osteoporosis.

F

Fallopian tube—The tube that carries the egg from the ovary to the uterus.

Femur—The large bone in the thigh whose upper end forms part of the hip joint.

Fibroids—Muscular tumors found in the uterus.

Flashes—See flushes. A term that describes a sudden sensation of intense warmth, which is caused by estrogen deficiency, in a menopausal woman.

Flexion exercises—This refers to exercises in which the movement of a joint causes the limbs above and below it to come together. In the case of the spine, this refers to exercises in which the spine bends forward from the waist and is rounded. These exercises are not recommended for women with osteoporosis.

Fluoride—The element fluorine combined with another element such as sodium. Sodium fluoride has been used in research studies as a potential treatment for osteo-porosis.

Flushes—See flashes. A term that describes a sudden sensation of intense warmth, which is caused by estrogen deficiency, in menopausal women.

Fosamax—The trade name for the new bis-phosphonate alendronate, which is manu-factured by Merck & Company. This drug is approved by the FDA for the treatment of osteoporosis.

Fracture—A break in a bone.

FSH—The abbreviation for follicle stimulat-ing hormone. A hormone that is made in a gland in the brain called the pituitary gland. This hormone stimulates the devel-opment of the follicle in the ovary, which will ultimately release an egg.

FDA—The abbreviation for the Food and Drug Administration.

G

Gonad—The medical term for the reproduc-tive glands of either a man or woman. The term can mean either ovaries or testes.

Gonadotropin—This refers to hormones that stimulate the production of estrogen in the ovaries or testosterone in the testes.

Gynecologist—A physician who specializes in the surgical treatment of diseases of a woman's reproductive system.

H

HDL—An abbreviation for high-density lipoprotein, which is a type of cholesterol not thought to be harmful.

Hip fracture—This refers to a fracture in the upper thigh bone or femur. Two types of hip fractures, cervical fractures and trochanteric fractures, are commonly seen in osteoporosis.

Hormone—A chemical substance produced in one organ of the body that controls or affects the functions of other organs in the body, like estrogen.

Hot flashes—See flushes. A feeling of intense warmth from within which can develop suddenly. It often awakens a woman at night. The cause is estrogen deficiency. This may be the earliest sign of menopause.

HRT—An abbreviation for hormone replace-ment therapy. The term implies the use of both estrogen and progesterone.

Hyperplasia—A condition in which the cells begin to grow abnormally. In some circum-stances, this is a precancerous condition.

Hypertension—The medical term for high blood pressure.

Hysterectomy—The surgical removal of the uterus or womb only. The term is often misused to mean the removal of the uterus and the ovaries.

I

Idiopathic—This term is often used to describe a disease in which the cause is unknown.

Impact-loading exercise—Exercise that causes an impact or jolt in the bones. Examples are jogging and skipping rope.

Isokinetic—A type of strength training or resistance exercise in which the speed of the movement against a resistance remains constant.

Isometric—A type of strength training or resistance exercise in which a muscle is tensed but does not actually contract. If you pushed as hard as you could against abrick wall, this would be isometric exercise.

Isotonic—A type of strength-training or resis-tance exercise in which the resistance against which the muscle contracts is con-stant but the muscle shortens and length-ens during the contraction.

L

Lactose—The type of sugar found in milk.

Lactose intolerance—A condition in which the milk sugar lactose causes diarrhea, abdominal pain, or bloating after being consumed. This condition often causes individuals to avoid dairy products, which contributes to calcium deficiency.

LDL—The abbreviation for low-density lipoprotcin. This is a type of cholesterol that may cause arteriosclerosis.

LH—The abbreviation for luteinizing hormone, a hormone produced in the pituitary gland in the brain that signals the ovary to release the egg.

Libido—The human sex drive.

Lumbar spine—The five individual bones or vertebrae in the lower back.

Luteal phase—This refers to the second half of the menstrual cycle after the egg has been released from the ovary.

M

Magnesium—A mineral necessary for proper growth and development of the skeleton.

Mammogram—An X-ray procedure to detect breast cancer.

Mead Johnson Laboratories—Manufacturers of Estrace, an oral estrogen tablet that has been approved by the FDA for the prevention of osteoporosis.

Medroxyprogesterone acetate—Often abbreviated MPA. This is a type of synthetic progesterone used in hormone replacement for postmenopausal women. It can also be used as a contraceptive and to control abnormal menstrual bleeding.

Menarche—The beginning of menstrual function.

Menopause—The failure of the ovaries, which causes estrogen deficiency and the loss of menstrual periods.

Merck—The pharmaceutical company that manufactures the new bisphosphonate alendronate, or Fosamax.

METS—This stands for metabolic equivalents. It is a measure of how hard the heart and lungs must work during an activity or exercise.

Miacalcin—The trade name for synthetic salmon calcitonin, which is manufactured by Sandoz Pharmaceuticals. Miacalcin is approved by the FDA for the treatment of osteoporosis and is available by prescription as either an injection or nasal spray.

Mrems—A measure of radiation exposure to a patient during an X-ray procedure. It is pronounced "milli-rems."

Musculoskeletal system—This refers to the muscles, ligaments, tendons, and bones of the human body.

N

Nephrolithiasis—The medical term for kidney stones.

O

Ogen The name for a form of oral estrogen replacement, which contains estrone, made by Upjohn Pharmaceuticals. Ogen is approved by the FDA for use in the prevention of osteoporosis.

Oophorectomy—See ovariectomy. The surgical removal of the ovaries.

Oral contraceptives—Birth control pills.

Os calcis—The medical term for the heel bone. Also called the calcaneus.

Osteoarthritis—A disease in which the lining of the joints is inflamed causing pain, swelling, and redness of the joints.

Osteomalacia—A disease of the bone in which the bone cannot properly incorporate calcium into the structure. The bones are often described as being soft.

Osteopenia—This term refers to a decrease in bone density that, although too low to be called normal, is not low enough to be considered osteoporotic.

Osteoporosis—A disease in which progressive bone loss causes the bones to become susceptible to breaking with little or no trauma.

Ovary—The female reproductive gland. Both estrogen and progesterone are made in this gland.

Ovariectomy—See oophorectomy. The medical term for the surgical removal of the ovaries.

Ovulation—The release of the egg by the ovary.

P

Partial hysterectomy—The surgical removal of the upper part of the uterus. The mouth of the uterus, or cervix, was not removed in this procedure, which is rarely performed now. The term is often misused to describe the removal of the entire uterus without the removal of the ovaries.

Patch, the—A slang term for the estrogen patch, Estraderm™ (estradiol transdermal system).

Peak bone mass—The maximum density of the bone, which is reached by young adulthood.

Pill, the—A slang term for oral contraceptive pills.

Pituitary gland—A small gland in the brain responsible for the production of several hormones, some of which control the production of estrogen and progesterone by the ovary.

Placebo—An inactive substance that is substituted for a medication in research studies. It is generally made to look like the active medication and used for comparison purposes in research.

Postmenopausal osteoporosis—Bone loss caused by estrogen deficiency that occurs at menopause. This is now called Type I osteoporosis.

Premarin—A form of oral estrogen replacement that contains conjugated equine estrogen. It is manufactured by Wyeth-Ayerst Pharmaceuticals and is approved by the FDA for use in the prevention and management of osteoporosis.

PremPhase—A new form of hormone replacement in which two rows of 7 tablets each of 0.625 mg of Premarin are provided on one card of a two card blister-pak. The second card contains two rows of 7 tablets each of a combination of 0.625 mg of Premarin and 5 mg of the brand of medroxyprogesterone called Cycrin. This preparation can be used by women electing to use standard cyclic hormone replacement therapy at menopause. This is manufactured by Wyeth-Ayerst.

PremPro—A new form of hormone replacement in which two rows of 7 tablets each are provided on two blister-pak cards. Each tablet contains 0.625 mg of Premarin and 2.5 mg of the brand of medroxyprogesterone called Cycrin. This preparation can be used by women electing to use the continuous combined form of hormone replacement therapy at menopause.

Primary osteoporosis—A category of osteoporosis that includes postmenopausal or Type I, senile or Type II, and idiopathic osteoporosis.

Proctor and Gamble Pharmaceuticals—Manufacturers of Didronel, a medication used in the treatment of Paget's disease and that is being investigated as a treatment for osteoporosis.

Progesterone—A hormone produced in the ovaries after ovulation occurs.

Progestins—Synthetic hormones that act similarly to progesterone.

Provera—The brand name for medroxyprogesterone acetate, which is manufactured by UpJohn Pharmaceuticals. This is a synthetic form of the natural female hormone progesterone and is therefore a progestin.

Puberty—The age at which the reproductive organs become developed.

Q

Quadriceps—The large muscle in the front of the thigh.

R

Radiation—Energy that is released by a source such as an X-ray tube.

Radius—A bone in the lower arm or forearm on the thumb side.

Reproductive organs—The ovaries in women and the testes in men.

Resistance exercise—See strength training. Exercise in which the muscle contracts or pulls against a weight or other resistance. This form of exercise was originally intended to increase muscle strength. It is also effective in improving bone strength.

Rhone-Poulenc Rorer Pharmaceuticals—Manufacturers of Calcimar, a synthetic salmon calcitonin used in the treatment of osteoporosis.

Rocaltrol—The trade name for the prescription form of 1,25 dihydroxy-vitamin D, which is manufactured by Roche Laboratories.

S

Salmon calcitonin—The calcitonin that is found in salmon. This type of calcitonin is more potent than human calcitonin. Synthetic salmon calcitonin is available as an injection or nasal spray for the treatment of osteoporosis.

Sandoz Pharmaceuticals—Manufacturers of Miacalcin, a synthetic salmon calcitonin used in the treatment of osteoporosis.

Secondary osteoporosis—A classification used to indicate that bone loss is the result of a disease other than estrogen deficiency or age.

Senile osteoporosis—Bone loss caused by factors attributed to aging, which includes calcium-deficient bone loss. This is now called Type II osteoporosis.

Single photon absorptiometry—A type of medical testing that uses a radioactive isotope to measure the bone density or bone mass in the wrist or heel. Often abbreviated as SPA.

Slow-release sodium fluoride—A new form of sodium fluoride that has been recommended for approval by the FDA for the treatment of osteoporosis.

Sodium fluoride—A salt of fluoride that contains sodium and fluorine. It has been used in research studies to treat advanced osteoporosis.

Steroids—Refers to many different chemical compounds that have the same basic chemical structure. Estrogen, testosterone, and cortisone are all steroids.

Strength training—Also called resistance training. This is exercise that utilizes weights or some other resistance against which the muscles push or pull.

Surgical menopause—Refers to the creation of menopause by the surgical removal of the ovaries in a woman who was still having menstrual periods.

T

Target heart rate—The heart rate to be reached during aerobic exercise to obtain heart benefits from exercising.

Testosterone—The male sex hormone.

Thiazides—A type of diuretic or fluid pill that is often used to treat high blood pressure or swelling. Thiazides may be useful in the treatment of osteoporosis by reducing the amount of calcium lost in the urine.

Thoracic spine—The 12 individual bones or vertebrae that make up the upper back from the base of the neck to just above the waist. Also called the dorsal spine.

Trace minerals—Minerals that are needed in very small amounts to maintain health. Examples are copper, manganese, and boron.

Transdermal—Refers to the delivery of medication through the skin.

Type I osteoporosis—A new name for postmenopausal osteoporosis.

Type II osteoporosis—A new name for senile osteoporosis.

U

Urethra—The tube that carries urine from the bladder out of the body.

Uterus—The medical term for the womb.

V

Vagina—The passageway from the uterus to the outside of the body.

Vertebra—The medical term for an individual bone in the spine. There are 7 vertebrae in the neck or cervical spine, 12 vertebrae in the upper back or thoracic spine, and 5 vertebrae in the lower back or lumbar spine.

W

Weight-bearing exercise—Exercise that requires the bones to support the weight of the body against gravity. Walking is weight-bearing exercise. Swimming is not considered a weight-bearing exercise.

Weight training—The use of dumbbells, barbells, or machines to increase muscle strength and endurance.

Withdrawal bleeding—Refers to uterine bleeding that occurs after hormone replacement is stopped or withdrawn.

Womb—The uterus.

Wyeth-Ayerst Pharmaceuticals—The company that makes Premarin, an oral estrogen tablet approved by the FDA for the prevention and management of osteoporosis.

X

X ray—electromagnetic energy that can pass through living tissue and expose a photographic plate.

Z

Zinc—A trace mineral. Deficiencies of zinc have been suggested as one cause of osteoporosis.

Index

193